God Bless -
Shelley
June 2001

Living with a Hog on my Back

The Story of a Multiple Sclerosis and Breast Cancer Survivor

Quincy Quay

Living with a Hog on my Back

The Story of a Multiple Sclerosis and Breast Cancer Survivor

Quincy Quay

ISBN: 1-891231-44-8

Library of Congress
Control Number:
2001089833

Word Association Publishers
205 Fifth Avenue
Tarentum, PA 15084
800-827-7903
www.wordassociation.com

Back Cover Photograph

Me, 8 years old

To Tom, who hasn't
deserted me

Acknowledgements

The most unfaltering, supportive and understanding person in my life is my husband, Tom, who has encouraged me to keep writing this story for the last three years. It was he who nonchalantly said, "You're always carrying a hog on your back," and thus gave me the story's unique title.

I give plenty of gratitude to my neighbor, Dr. Frank Bontempo, who gave my—needs lots of work—draft its first critique.

Much credit goes to Clark Thomas, senior editor (retired), with the Pittsburgh Post-Gazette, for his suggestions. I was led by his clear-sighted and intuitive direction.

Great appreciation goes to my cousin, Robert J. Robinson, for his extraordinary and marvelous photographs. The lamenting letter he shared with me wonderfully fits into my story.

I am grateful to David Fligger, who bestowed to me the photographs of Winifred Lynch and the Lynch family.

The portrait of Major Alexander Hanna is courtesy Michael P. Connelly. My story title is a take-off from Michael's dramatic tale of Alexander.

The back cover photo was bestowed to me courtesy of Robert Copenhaver.

I give thanks to my family and Tom's family; for all the enduring love and support a person could want. I'm especially grateful to my cousin, Robert J. Robinson, for his encouragement, love and guidance. Special thanks to my friend and confidante, Mary Palmer, for her love and encourgement, and special thanks to my friend, Mary Nicklow, for her love and generosity.

And, a great appreciation to my tremendous and caring doctors.

CONTENTS

Foreword

One day in 1993, shortly after suffering a cerebral hemorrhage, I sat pondering family memories, and the genealogy that I'd left untouched since the 1970's. For some reason, there was a nagging childhood incident that I wanted to investigate. It seemed my soul was searching for something that wasn't apparent, at least, until now. What clue could my family history hold for me—in coping with unmerciful difficulties—and would I uncover a trace of my strong spirit in them? What memories triggered that thought pattern? And, what ability did I grasp from my early upbringing, in making life choices, in shaping how I perceive the world?

We all carry a "hog on our back" at one time or another in life. All of us eventually have our burdens or times of illness or death of loved ones, and some of us even carry guilt throughout our lives.

My unusual inspirational tale may generate possibility, or enlightenment, or perhaps encouragement for those seeking God. I now realize that writing the highlights of my life has unbound and set me free. I hope it will amaze, astound and shock others into reexamining their purpose for being here. Is our life just a coincidence or does it follow a pre-destined pattern?

Ancestors of Michele Quay Nicklow

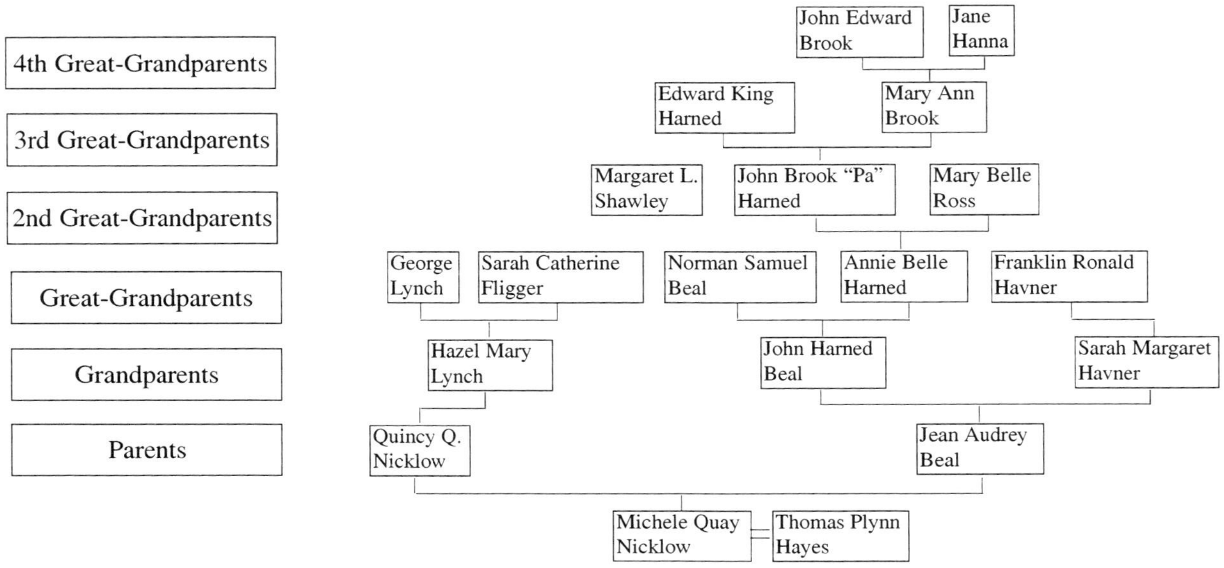

It don't matter where you bury me,
I'll be home and I'll be free.
It don't matter where I lay,
All my tears be washed away.
(Julie Miller)

1

On July 4th, 1952, I entered the world with a "bang." I was my father's daughter, and was given his middle name Quay. A great uncle was to call me a "firecracker" and "pistol" of a child. Little did I know the pistol was loaded, waiting to go off. Like a boisterous, bucking bronco, wildly anxious to be released from its stall, I was excitable and energetic.

From the beginning I was branded like a mark of birth. Born a month early, and weighing a frail three pounds and four ounces, I was incubated and neglected in the old frame hospital where I was born. I was horribly allergic to milk. Eczema all over, with constant scratching and wailing—what a miserable, suffering mess I was. When mom brought me home, she clipped my nails, and tried mittens to keep me from maiming myself. At her wits' end, she pinned my hands down with the covers to stop the incessant clawing.

Soon, Mom visited old Dr. Curr, who prescribed raw milk and said, "Skim the cream."

I grew fat and happy.

It's January 1956, and I'm sitting on the floor. I look up to see tall strange people standing in dark clothing. I look to my right, where the sun is streaming in. I guess I'm drawn to the sun's rays on the floor, the only bright spot, in a dark, somber room. I wanted to go out and play. It was a strange scene indeed, and I might have even taken a peak at my now deceased maternal great grandfather, Franklin Havner, who was laid-out in his home. My younger cousin took one look at him and ran out of the house. He wouldn't go back in.

I'd always held this faint image, but didn't think it real until my mother spoke of his funeral, years later. Now, years subsequent, I asked my grandma, Margaret Havner, if I'd been at her pa's funeral.

"Yes," she said, "you were there, crawling on the floor, playing."

Memory plays tricks, surely; still, I can accurately place the floor plan from where I sat. Memories intertwine with surreal images of dreams. Anyway, I believe this to be my first recollection, and I guess you could say it helped prepare me for what lay ahead.

My mother's family is talkative, direct and expressive. Their anger is clearly emphatic. In contrast, Dad's siblings are soft spoken and quiet. Less communication here, and especially so after their father up and left the family. I have child–like questions, but Father always says, "Grandpa is dead."

Then one evening the forbidden happens at the dinner table.

"If he's dead why haven't I seen his grave?" I innocently asked.

The table grows quiet. Grandma Hazel Lynch, sitting across from me, looks at Dad, then puts her head down and mumbles.

Later, I'm told he had taken their savings, and run off to California, years earlier. Dad, with his brothers and sisters, became resourceful.

The Mennonites in my small hometown of Scottdale, Pennsylvania—who are my distant cousins—started a publishing house. I went to school with their children. One of Dad's friends was Mennonite, and it was to his house my parents and I gathered for a game of cards one night.

Snacks were brought out, including Brazil nuts. I ate one and immediately went into the throes of an explosive anaphylactic reaction, that transported me into a frightening world. I entered the midst of giant hives and angioedema, barely able to breathe. I began to drown in their inflammation. I remember pulling at my mother's clothes while she held me in her lap. We rushed home, where the family physician was waiting for us.

I've been told I have an extraordinarily resolute way about me. It probably stems from the traumatic experiences of my infancy, and that hazy funeral, and later, the death of my father, Quincy Quay Nicklow.

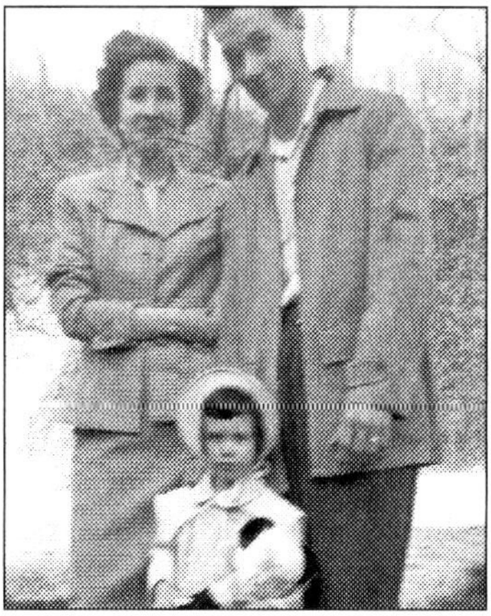

My parents and I at Easter, circa 1956.

My mom, Audrey Beal, showed courage and strength when he died. He suffered a cerebral hemorrhage, due to a ruptured aneurysm, around Thanksgiving. After a lengthy operation, he passed away January 19, 1967. He never woke up and I was fourteen years old.

When I was a child, one of my bedroom windows faced the entrance to the town's graveyard, with its iron–gate and worn, blackened tombstones. On a warm summer's night, I might spy Harlem, the town character, hunched over his wheelbarrow, ambling along the moonlit graveyard. That was spooky to a kid.

My father dies, in my 14th year, a ray of sun in a dark room, a Grandfather not dead, not buried, and Harlem's bent, dark, shadowy frame in the night. This was some of my childhood. And, it was all welling to a certain, imminent fate.

For over the last twelve years, it's as if I've been thrown over an apex by some scathing, murderous mob, left only to hobble down a dimly lit, nightmarish road. With no way station or solace in sight, I'm forced to lay out the playing cards I carry in my hand. Is it God who controls the "laying of the hands"?

"An Ancient Rockshelter And A 60 Foot Cross"

2

Untamed energy and erratic behavior marked my early childhood. It affected my ability to concentrate—I was a constant daydreamer—and learn in school. I was unpredictable, shy and introverted. In the 3rd grade, I was frightened of the teacher who smacked her students. She told my mother I was stupid.

In high school I did well in English, my favorite subject. Other curiosities and mysteries would, however, beckon and pull at me: primarily anything that dealt with the past. I find nothing more fun than going through some person's cluttered, dusty attic, or rooting through the pages of an old archive.

Accepted at Penn State University, I majored in anthropology. I almost chose English for my major, but I went with my heart and chose anthropology instead. I was tired of tearing apart every book I read, which took away the enjoyment of reading. Besides, anthropology/archaeology was more of a challenge and sounded like fun. My college major eventually led me to delve into my ancestry; later, both would come in handy for "digging" up answers to my medical questions.

Jimmy Watson, a good friend of my maternal grandfather, John Beal, sparked my initial interest in archaeology. After dinner, we'd all sit around drinking coffee and eating dessert, anticipating Jimmy's tales of Amazon expeditions and Mayan archeological ruins. He was in the lumber business. A short man with beady, watery eyes, he always wore a safari hat. I was an enthralled listener.

In the summer of 1971, between my freshman and sophomore year, I registered for a field course in archaeology, at the California University, in California, Pennsylvania. The excavation of an early inn, located along historic Route 40—America's first toll road—was part of the study, along with a Monongahela (Native American) Village located near Grindstone, in Fayette County.

Early one morning, while driving to the inn, I had quite a scare. Sudden dizziness made me pull off to the side of the road. It quickly dissipated, but I sat there a while until I was sure.

Another morning, I excitedly leapt out of bed to get dressed for the dig, when a wave of vertigo threw me off balance. Since I always had low blood pressure this could have explained the episode.

Another time, during the early 70's, I felt a foot go numb while riding in the car with Mom. She made the comment that perhaps I had pinched a nerve in my back. The foot numbness went away after visits to a chiropractor.

A couple of years later, now at the main campus of Penn State, I had a miniscule incident of slurred speech while talking on the telephone. In another incident, a book I had picked up by its binding just suddenly dropped out of my hand. These two minor events, even though they were bizarre, were momentary, and never happened to me again while I was in college.

I still had physical education courses to take while at the main campus. Innocuous signs of lassitude began showing up in the last of these PE classes. In order to graduate I had to pass a swim test; so, swimming became one of my final courses. Being so thin, I didn't have the stamina, nor the right body type needed to be a swimmer, but I still enjoyed it.

Having good coordination, my gymnast friend, Peggy, encouraged me to sign up for gymnastics. Now I was really out of the water. I lacked the physical strength need for strenuous athletics, and it was soon after that I began dragging one leg. I also developed a backache. Peggy thought that perhaps I did something to my back; so, she took me to see her chiropractor.

Even though the PE classes I took during my junior and senior year were tasking, I never thought to link the weakness I was experiencing to my physical activity. Anytime I did the "out of the ordinary," my body would relay another signal to lay more foundation in a mysterious disease. I was completely ignorant of it all.

I blamed my general lassitude, the leg dragging, and my speech and book incident on everything at college: maybe I was studying too hard, maybe I needed vitamins, maybe I didn't like the winters there, or maybe I didn't like the large campus. The "real" fatigue would come years later.

Just what good is a Bachelor of Arts in Anthropology? Not much, I already knew, when I graduated in 1974. For the next two years, until I decided what to do the rest of my life, I lived with my mother in her hometown of Connellsville. I took a couple of waitress jobs for a time. For interest outside of work, I joined a local historical society, and began a genealogy project.

It was about 1975, that another unnatural phenomena happened to me. It was in a motel swimming pool in Ohio. I struggled to swim to the other end of the pool. When I pushed myself out of the pool, and sat on the edge, I grew quite weak with numbness. While sitting there, I made a chilling comment to my mom about the oddness of the moment.

A little while after this episode, I heard a neat talk that rescued me from an unproductive life. Early in the spring of 1976, I attended a local historical society event and heard a guest speaker, from the University of Pittsburgh, give a lecture on an obscure archaeological site called the "Meadowcroft Rockshelter." The grand crusade of its adventure lured me in and I eagerly volunteered for the dig.

The shelter is perched on a steep hill about 40 miles west of Pittsburgh. The closer you get to the shelter, the more treacherous the road becomes. A dangerous "S" curve, a bridge over Cross Creek, and there you are.

If you stand in the middle of Cross Creek—the shelter resides on its north, 15.06 m above the creek—and look up you would see it's roughly oriented east west, with a southern exposure. "The area protected by the extant overhang is 65 m2 while the overhang itself is some 13 m above the modern surface of the site."

The University of Pittsburgh recorded the site in 1968. Their Archaeological Research Program, from the Department of Anthropology, left it untouched until the spring of 1973, when they were looking for a field school site. They "dug in."

At first sight, the shelter's magnificent jutting overhang and two fallen blocks—that lay east and west on the perimeters—rightly impress you. When these blocks were originally in situ (part of the overhang), the shelter was three or four times larger than it is today.

Next came a platform entryway that housed tools, a telephone and a computer—all of which looked "jarringly out of place in a cave." By the time I was there, a guard tent and a picnic table (at times leaning precariously) completed the scene. James Adovasio says, "We've recovered nearly 3 1/2 million objects here." And: "We removed 130 metric tons of soil, digging with nothing larger than trowels. Sometimes a living floor was thinner than a trowel; then we dug with razor blades."

Today, years after my 1976 experience, the rockshelter is still on the cutting edge of man's first waves of migration into North America. New data is pushing the arrival time of the early Americans, back further and further, "into exciting disarray," leading archaeologist to reexamine old sites.

The rockshelter's many well-documented radiocarbon dates of 10,900-12,950 BP (before present), just fuels argumentation, with the latest archaeological discoveries of Kennewick Man, "a well-preserved, 9,500-year-old human skeleton found in Washington State in 1996, Nevada's Spirit Cave Man, Idaho's Buhl Woman and Brazil's Luzia. Monte Verde, a site in Chile, has credible evidence dating back 14,500 years." (Nova's, February 15, 2000, Mystery of the First Americans.)

On the first May mountain night of my excavating adventure, it was so cold that the skeleton crew and I sat huddled around a Coleman lantern, and passed around a bottle of whiskey to keep warm. The mobile home, whose floor we sat on, was being used for the project.

It's not difficult to drum up romantic notions about the place. The rockshelter is a beautiful spot, especially on a crisp early morning, when you can see your breath, and all is still and quiet. Before excavation started on these cold mornings, we'd light a fire on our choice rock slab. Here, we'd stand around a bit, or sit on our haunches looking out over the creek, drinking coffee to keep warm. During such moments, I often wondered what thoughts the ancient inhabitants held, gazing out over the same scene.

The witty and wild crew was terrific fun– at all times. Frank constantly entertained us with his funny endless stories. Augie was the nice guy who got saddled with all the carpentry jobs. Andie's family had fled Hungary when she was two years of age. She was the most free-spirited one of the group. The last I heard, Andie has her doctorate degree and three children. Rhonda was always up at camp, sitting in the old mine house we used, drafting complex basketry. Joel, a laid-back University of Texas professor, from San Antonio, brought his wife, baby and black lab, Jasper. Jasper loved Cross Creek.

Routine cleanup at the dig took at least an hour, and was a top priority because of contamination. Banana brushes were used to sweep the entire site, including the wooden steps down to the road. The following year, an electric shop vacuum would be used inside the shelter. Meals were cooked in the convenient old house that sat above the shelter. At one time it was used as a coal mine office. Two refrigerators and two stoves were there for our use, and the mine office safe was our pantry. The place was kept spotlessly clean by scrubbing the linoleum floor every night (among other chores), including under the refrigerators.

And we kept "ourselves" clean by showering at a local golf course. The first time I drove my 4-cylinder Chevy Vega to get the anticipated shower, I got lost and ended up in a cemetery. As I crested a hill, I looked straight across at another ridge. There stood a huge cross. I was stunned for a moment.

I never mentioned the incident back in camp, but knew it happened to be the Jumonville Cross. Located high on Chestnut Ridge, it sits above a Methodist Church camp, in southwestern Pennsylvania.

The tall, sturdy steel cross was named after Ensign Joseph Coulon de Villiers, the Sieur de Jumonville—the French officer and commander who was killed, on May 28, 1754, by George Washington and his men.

Since 1950, a steel cross, 60 feet high, has stood on a concrete base six feet tall on Dunbar's Knob, which itself is 2,480 feet above sea level. On a clear day the mountaintop boasts a view of three states and seven counties with sights up to 50 miles away. At night it is bathed in glowing spotlights, shining as a beacon of hope and inspiration to all that see it far above the dark silhouette of the Appalachian Mountains.

A foundation consisting of 183 tons of concrete had to be constructed. Then, the main shaft of the cross, weighing approximately 47,000 pounds, had to be hauled to the mountaintop site, after cutting a road up the back side of the mountain. The arms, projecting 12 feet on each side of the main shaft, were brought in separately and the entire structure was securely welded together.

Because of its exposed location, the bracing of the structure had to be thorough, but all bracing is inside the clean-cut steel surface of the cross. The completed structure will withstand winds of 100 miles an hour and the torsion that might be developed by a whirlwind. (Courtesy LR Beatty)

Just about every night it was social time at Lou's a small local bar. John Denver's "Country Roads" was our jukebox theme song, and soon we began to dominate the scene. We got so familiar at the bar that James (head instructor) began to help himself to pitchers of beer and food for us. You could do the bar scene a few nights in a row, then you had to stay in recovery, back at camp, at least one night a week.

During the '76 dig season, the crew held a big July 4th cookout in the picnic pavilion of the historical Meadowcroft Village (which sits above the shelter). That night they gave me a surprise 24th birthday cake that Dave had baked earlier. Later we trooped over to Lou's, where I was served shots of tequila. Someone else would drive my car back to camp that night.

It was times like these that I would ask Joel about any upcoming archaeology projects that I could do next.

"In the fall," he said, "there's going to be a surface survey in southern New Mexico."

It was to be through Joel's department, the Center for Archaeological Research, at the University of Texas. It would be there that I journeyed next.

It had been a heady, jubilant time for me at Meadowcroft and no strange, unexplainable dizziness, speech impediments or numbness or fatigue showed up during that May to August of 1976, like it had in the past. Perhaps I was under the protection of that cross.

Except, I specifically recall feeling lousy, the one rainy day I spent working in the dig's temporary lab, which had been setup in someone's garage. Naturally, anyone can have a bad day or feel blue, especially on a miserable day. So I forgot about it.

But there must having been something going on before that trip to New Mexico, in October, because I made an appointment with a physician in my former hometown of Scottdale. I wasn't feeling quite right. I remember explaining my misgivings to the doctor. I blamed it on my allergies and he gave me an injection for them. I soon felt better and my feeling vaguely out-of-sorts slipped away.

MS is a very insidious disease.

3

In October of 76, I flew to San Antonio toting a brand new, army green duffel bag and knapsack. I stayed with Joel and his family for a couple of days, until the small University of Texas survey crew and I headed west, towards El Paso. The Bureau of Land Management, under terms of contract (YA-512-RFP6-80) with the archaeological center, was to fund the survey, calling it the "Radium Springs Archaeological Project."

The Radium Springs survey was commenced by the BLM, because they wanted a statistical representation of cultural evidence, from all the areas that they owned in southern New Mexico. It was to be included in their upcoming and complete account of the "Radium Springs Geothermal Leasing Environmental Analysis Record." Our fieldwork would provide the BLM with the valid random statistics they required for showing "cultural resource densities within various environmental zones in the project area."

The focus of the survey was a desolate region called the Jornada del Muerto. It lies between the Caballo and San Andres Mountains. The San Andres, to the east, were outside our range. The White Sands Missile Range lay over the San Andres. The intense survey would take approximately two months to complete.

A computer randomly selected samples, for our required contract's 32 square mile sections, to be surveyed. Our crew accomplished this and more, tacking on an extra section, and recording six important sites that lay outside the boundaries of the survey. 30 of our 33 sections were located through the use of USGS or U.S. Geological Survey section markers.

Our crew's transportation, to each mapped section, was a rugged university vehicle with a wench on the front bumper in case we hit rough territory.

While walking the rugged terrain we carried long cane poles, topped with orange plastic flags, to stay inline, at least 50 meters apart. Some of us carried maps, cameras, compasses and CB radio transmitters, and we all carried a police whistle, paper bags and coding forms for recording data. Along the way, we might encounter hazardous deep arroyos, where we had to pull each other. On one occasion, we had to leave the area while White Sands did one of its routine missile launches.

A good-natured local rancher and his wife were on the project payroll (since they knew the territory well), working a day ahead of us, staking out each square mile for us to tack. We camped on their ranch for a spell, and engaged our host and hostess to cook our meals in their homey, warm two–room cabin. We used water from their cistern for washing.

There were a lot of uneventful moments in our daily excursions, but sometimes we got out of sync and were separated. One day, Steve, our group leader, was nowhere to be found. While the rest of us stood together for a break, we heard a yapping in the distance. Soon, a disgusted Steve appeared, dragging his pole behind him. He had entered coyote den territory.

At night, we all sat around a campfire, gazing up at endless stars, and listening to coyote symphonies. My most memorable experience, even though it was quite cold at night, was taking a bath in a large wash tub and looking up at those endless stars.

During the day, the sunlight was radiant and intense. Since there was little pollution or humidity, desert colors shown brilliantly. We could see the town of Truth or Consequences, glistening, miles away in the distance. What an exhilarating experience. What would I discover today?

A retired army colonel, working on his master's degree, headed the project. Every morning we arose to a bugle call and an army song.

We sometimes arose to snow in our tents, and on one such morning I found a nice stiff rat in mine. I picked up the disgusting varmint by the tail and threw it out of the tent. The guys had stashed it in my snowy abode, waiting for the scream that never happened.

Another day, our rancher host threw an old, diffused missile section into the vehicle where the colonel was siting. He quickly got out.

Our surface survey yielded pottery and lithic artifacts including projectile points, scrapers and drills of gray chert. Monos and metates, for grinding grain, were rare in this semi-desert region. The distinctive mineral malachite was often found. Native Americans used it for ornamental and jewelry decoration.

Historically, the Jornada del Muerto region of New Mexico was the home of the Mescalero Apache. The Jornada del Muerto is a "ninety-mile stretch of waterless desert—a short cut which saved distance, but cost many lives, since the Native Americans could lurk in the mountains and pounce on their victims without warning. So many travelers were killed that this particular stretch was known as the Jornada del Muerto-the day's journey of the dead man (Sonnichscn 1958:49)" Today, it's still known as the "journey of death" or the "journey of the dead."

By accident—we were hunting for a section marker—we came across a pottery bowl holding a cache of turquoise beads. Dubbed the "High Lonesome Bead Cache," it lay outside of the survey range, along the western foothills of the San Andres. Its significance was never to be revealed. We could only conclude that it had been buried, but forgotten by its native owner. We came upon an abandoned ranch and windmill near the bead cache, with a sign that read, "High Lonesome:" hence the name of the site.

The crew and I worked extended hours and completed the project in record time. It enabled us to spend a long weekend in Juarez, Mexico. We went to an indoor market where we browsed over goods displayed in a quiet museum like atmosphere. This way we weren't constantly hassled by pushy venders.

While at the museum, we made the mistake of trusting one crewmember who had lived in Mexico, for a period. He told the taxi driver to wait at the entrance for us. We just sort of looked at him, and then at each other, and shrugged our shoulders, as if to say, "Guess he knows what he's doing."

When we came out, three hours later, the tab was outrageous.

Before we ran for the border, the guys bought and loaded us girls up with cheap liquor. Oh, no, that's not what I meant. They had us girls carrying at least two bottles each when we crossed over the border.

At the survey's end I flew home, via Albuquerque, with a stop over at the O'Hara Airport in Chicago. At the O'Hara (I thought "cultural shock" was just a silly anthropological term) I stood gazing in amazement, wondering where everyone was rushing. After all, I had been lost in the "journey of death" for four weeks.

During my last days in New Mexico, before my scheduled flight home, I stayed for a couple of days with my ranch host's son and his family, in their three-room house. I remember lying awake in the morning without much pep, even though I'd always been an enthusiastic morning person.

I spent the winter back home in Connellsville, where I began to be plagued with constipation—a common complaint of MS patients. I tried to fix it with laxatives.

I later learned that for some MS patients, this is how their symptoms progressed—deceptively, over a long period of time, or their symptoms would go into remission for a spell, after periodic attacks. For others, acute attacks give a clear sign of real illness. Luckily for some, their MS appears to halt.

My next dig would be a premonition of what was to come.

4

The next spring I made arrangements to go back to Meadowcroft, under the auspices of a field credit course. However, I wasn't satisfied with the year's dig season because I was relegated to the sifting screens—perhaps, because I wasn't a fulltime University of Pittsburgh student.

I was at Meadowcroft for only a short while, when a salaried archaeology position with Boston University, in Boston, came along. My job title was to be "Technical Staff Assistant." There would be two instructors.

The 1977 summer project was the excavation of an early glass factory, located upon the hilltop of a wooded area in Temple Township, Hillsborough County, in southern New Hampshire. BU conducted the dig from 1975 to 1978.

The glass factory was one of only a hand full of 18th-century industrial sites. Robert Hewes founded the Temple Glass Factory, which was in operation from 1780 to 1782. It marked the beginning of glass making in New Hampshire—using Hessian mercenaries, from the British Army, to manufacture the early bottles. Also, there were early attempts at making crude window-glass.

This experience would prove to be most difficult excavating project I was to be involved with. We had to drag cumbersome gear up to the site and back every day: photographic equipment, a transit, notebooks and a cooler that contained our lunch.

My back became so stiff from carrying the loads that I slid out of bed every morning, rather than bending my back. This was hard on a person of small stature who weighed only 90 lbs.

The constipation I had been dealing with back home became worse. I ignored it, deciding that back strain from heavy lifting caused it.

The excavation setup was much different from Meadowcroft. We ate and slept indoors, in a big old inn located a few miles outside the quaint historical town of Peterborough. A barn next to the inn housed a large number of bats. It would become very bat-like at night.

The university, who owned the two buildings, was conducting scientific research on the barn bats. A few of these bats would always manage to wonder into the inn. We ate our meals on a long slab of a table in the large added sunroom. Every day we had to scrub the table down because of bat dung.

Everything that could go wrong seemed to go wrong in New Hampshire. It started the first weekend I was there. Before the field school even began, the instructor who brought us there had up and left for the weekend, leaving me, and two other girls, with out a vehicle. Since there was no food in the pantry, we had to hike a long distance into the village for the groceries we needed. On the walk back to the inn, I kept zigzagging all over the road, and by the time we returned I was worn out.

I and some of the crew got really perturbed when one of the professors decided to invite a colleague and his field school students for a weekend of fun at our camp. He never bothered to confer with us before hand, and we had to feed and entertain rude people who never bothered to raise a hand.

After the dig ended, the crew was invited to the same instructor's apartment for a little partying. At the same time, the digs other instructor, Ben, was working in the anthropology lab down the street.

Meanwhile, a couple of guys went out and came back to the apartment with alcoholic beverages and squirt guns. Now, it was a very hot day, and our host and hostess had no air conditioning. The squirt guns were a great way to stay cool and have fun. Then someone decided that we should venture down the street and ambush dour Ben.

Once inside the old brick anthropology building we all found a niche to hide. Guessing something was up; Ben went looking, and found me first, hiding behind a door. Red faced and in a rage, he grabbed the toy gun out of my hand and wrenched my arm in the process.

Next, into the hall, he attacked a young fellow who had been hanging around with a girl he had wanted. A couple of guys pulled him off. I guess we conceded that "the party was over."

When the field season was over, at the end of August, Mom and her friend picked me up at the Pittsburgh Airport. We stopped to eat at a restaurant, on the way home to Connellsville. Sitting at the table, I remember wondering why I was in such a dark mood. I should be excited, talking about my trip. Severe constipation and a stiff back made me irritable.

So, at home that fall of '77, I began to focus on the now overt constipation, which made me feel distressed and miserable. I tried not to abuse laxatives. I spent a lot of time in the bathroom.

It's hard for me to remember those sly body signals of the 70's, but now that I look back, the MS attributes were there. Lack of overt signs can make it difficult for doctors to confirm MS.

In September, my grandparents, my mom and I drove to Silver Springs, Maryland to visit Mom's sister, Patti and her family. Still having bowel problems I didn't sleep well there. I started taking potent vitamins and eating wheat germ. The wheat germ gave me an itchy rash.

That winter, I visited my OBGYN because I had a bladder infection—another red flag for MS.

I had never had a bladder infection before. Interestingly, my Aunt Patti had a kidney removed around that same time. She had suffered with bladder infections since she was a child, later finding out that she had been born with a diseased kidney. Her dad, who is my granddad, John Beal, also had had a kidney removed some years back.

This led me to believe that I'd inherited a predisposition to urology problems, which is how I now began to explain my bladder difficulty. In gripping pain one night—while Mom was in Silver Spring caring for my Aunt Patti, after her operation—I realized I must have passed a kidney stone. I went to see a faceless doctor who surmised that I'd had had a stone.

In the meantime, I made plans to move to Pittsburgh and go back to school for graduate studies. Mom didn't want me to leave home— she and I were very close—but what opportunity did I have in the small town of Connellsville, where many of the young people left?

5

In the early spring of 1978, I started classes at the University of Pittsburgh, taking nine graduate credits. The semester proved pretty tough. First, I'd been out of school for four years. Second, walking on deep snow-covered sidewalks became exhausting, especially since I was always lugging weighty books of various archaeological research. I held the same books while I stood on a crowded bus, riding out to the campus from downtown Pittsburgh. Since I sold my Vega, and wasn't living on campus, I had to catch two buses– one to town (from the room I rented) and another out to Pitt. I became burned out.

I signed up for three courses, each from different sub-fields of anthropology: Old and New World Monkeys, European Archaeology and native, Southeastern U.S. Cultural Anthropology.

The physical anthropology "monkey" course caused me the most havoc. So much detail I didn't know what I should know. I was sure you had to be an anatomist. The professor focused on her night-monkey study, so the class became well versed in all their little details. With her down jacket on, the instructor bore a distinct resemblance to the ape world. Rumor had it that her night–monkey project was a sham; after all, no one ever actually SAW one of her elusive monkeys.

Class grades went downhill, including mine, with each exam. By the last, everyone was shaking his or her head. I was luckier than some students who would be unable to graduate after the spring semester was over.

Even though I enjoyed the European archaeology class, it turned out to be a problem for me, too. The flighty instructor kept changing the course requirements. "You can do three small papers," or the next day it would be, "You can do one big paper."

He vacillated around so much, that I lost the precious time required for completing a decent paper. Asking questions I'd only get vague answers. I went through the whole course never really figuring out what he preferred, or what sparked his interest, but I made it through OK.

Language was another challenge, because all those European archaeology journals have to be translated. I was totally unprepared to jump into a foreign language, but so were the other students in the class. So there was a mad scramble for the British Isles Monolithic Culture that included Stonehenge. I lost.

I became engrossed in the Southeastern anthropology class. I did well in the course, after writing a historical comparison between the white man's version—about the demise of the Native American—and what the Native Americans themselves said happened. I used two books as sources: Mari Sandoz's *Crazy Horse, and The Long Death*: *The Last Days of the Plains Indians* by Ralph Andrist.

After the semester was over I took the graduate records examination or GRE. In the meantime, I signed up for a summer archeological course with Pitt. Even thought the dig wasn't like the in-house Meadowcroft Rockshelter, I was still counting on being at the dig most of the time; so hurriedly, and without care, I rented an apartment on the Pitt campus. Located on the same street, and very near the old anthropology building, its one occupant was looking for two people.

But Pitt felt, and rightly so, that since I wasn't a full-time student, I shouldn't get first pick to participate in the excavation. So, when the dig fell through, I was stuck with two roommates I didn't know.

I discovered that young, troubled, Edie's parents had thrown her out of the house. We shared a bedroom. Soon she decided her boyfriend should be her bedmate, and suggested I move out and move in with a guy I'd been dating.

Disgusted, I went looking for a better situation. When I found better-adjusted roommates, I up and left. Then I called the apartment managers and told them why I wouldn't be paying my next month's rent.

One day Edie telephones me at my temporary bar/restaurant job and says I left a jacket behind. Naïvely and stupidly, I went back to the apartment. I knocked on the door.

Answering, Edie suddenly grabs me around the throat, and pushes me backwards, into a chair.

"You bitch!" she screamed, while holding my throat and slapping my face.

I put my feet up, trying to push her away.

"No," I said. "You've got it all wrong. You're the bitch!"

She just slapped harder.

The other roommate pulled her off me, and I escaped down the stairs and out the door onto the grimy street.

My new roommates, Barbara, Diane and Carol were lively commercial art students, up all hours, airbrushing, while I stepped over their latest project. They were fairly mature, and I was glad their parents hadn't thrown them out because of any rebelliousness.

A new town, a new apartment...a new gynecologist. It was summer 1978, and I began having bladder troubles that sent me to the bathroom too many times at night.

"We have to find out why you keep getting bladder infections," the female gynecologist said.

But nothing was done.

I hammered at the doctor until she finally set up an exploratory examination or a laparoscopy of my pelvic organs. It's done by inserting a laparoscope through the abdominal wall.

Before surgery, I was given pre-op instructions by the doctor's office. But somehow there was a mix-up and a resulting confusion, over the preparation procedures involving food and drink. They said I hadn't followed the rules. They operated anyway.

After my surgery as a short-stay patient the nurses couldn't wake me up. (Uncommon sleepiness can be early sign of a troubled nervous system.) It was five or six o'clock, closing time, when the nurses woke me up and I had to leave. The medical staff wouldn't let me take a bus home, so I telephoned a great aunt and uncle in a Pittsburgh suburb, and they picked me up and took me back to my apartment.

The results of the surgery showed a mild case of endometriosis, and I was put on oral contraceptives for six months.

Endometriosis occurs when normal tissue grows beyond the uterus.

"Tissue similar to the lining of the uterus takes hold elsewhere in your body. The misplaced tissue responds to hormones the way the uterine lining does, with a buildup of tissue followed by

shedding. This tissue has no natural exit route from the body, however, and can lead to pain and inflammation in the pelvic regions including the abdomen, ovaries, bladder and bowel."

This was really it. Now I had the absolute answer to my bladder and bowel miseries.

I joined in the social life of my newfound roommates. With Barbara, her boyfriend and his church group I went for a night of outdoor ice-skating, where I soon realized I was an absolute "failure on ice," with ankles so weak I couldn't balance. I had been a good skater in my teen years. Confused and mad, because of the surprising weakness, I took it out on the fellow who was my date. Playing volleyball was something else the church group did once a month, but I had no energy for that either.

Upon advice from Aunt Patti, I went to see an internist.

He asked me, "What's the problem?"

"I've been getting backaches," I said. (How do you describe obscure problems?)

Then he asked me, "Whom did you inherit your crooked back from?"

I said, "I don't know."

He recommended wearing a back brace during physical activity, and I started wearing one during the church volleyball games.

I was getting a little irate, because I started to realize that some of the physicians, I saw during this period, felt they were dealing with a hypochondriac, inferring that it was "all in my head." Of course they just didn't know.

Since I was still having trouble with my bowels, I made an appointment with a gastroenterologist at a local clinic—another "all in my head" doctor, it turns out.

"Try eating right," he disgustedly said, after my sigmoidoscopic exam. Without direct medical evidence I was getting all sorts of uninviting comment.

In the meantime, I received my GRE results, which weren't the best, but I applied for graduate school anyway. Later, I received a departmental letter extolling a non-acceptance. They suggested I complete another semester. Since I didn't have any more funds for the moment, I quickly took a downtown accounting job in a men's clothing store, after quitting my part time, temporary bar/restaurant job.

Shortly after I received the GRE notice, I stopped in the anthropology department. While I sat talking to the receptionist she got a phone call and was called away. The temptation was too much. I got up and peeked into the files to see what was written about my non-acceptance. Of the three judges, one said "yes" and two said "no."

After working at the clothing store for a short while, I finally landed a clerical job in the Pittsburgh branch of the Insurance Services Office (ISO).

It was not long after, in August of 1979, that I met my future husband, Tom. He immediately reminded me of my nature-loving granddad, John Beal. My heart told me that the two of us belonged together and we were married on January 5th, 1980.

6

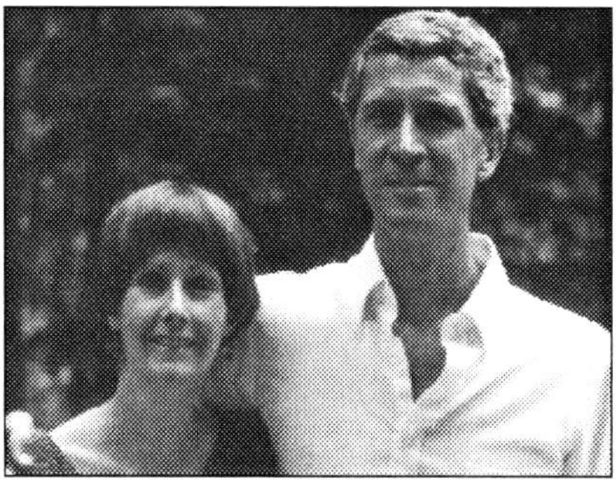

Tom and me

We met in a local, Pitt campus, restaurant and bar. Like me, Tom had a slim build, with dark hair and blue eyes. He said he grew up in Washington County, Pennsylvania. I told him about the Meadowcroft Rockshelter—situated on land owned by one Albert Miller—in Washington County.

Then, he told me he'd worked at the Meadowland's Trotter Racetrack (which was operated by Albert's brother) when he was a teenager. With sleek horses raring to go, he didn't like their wild behavior.

Tom and I were connected even before we met because Tom's parents knew Albert's brother, Delvin. They had owned and raced a couple of trotters, at The Meadowlands, during the early 70's.

Tom is a genuinely thoughtful guy. Like his mother, Tom's a sympathetic listener and a loyal person, who defends the underdog. He is the peacemaker, smoothing over problems between people.

Tom's background was similar to mine except that he had a younger brother and sister. Jay, two years younger, was diagnosed with diabetes at the age of fourteen. With his gregarious personality (opposite Tom's) he went on to become a heavy equipment salesman like his father.

Carla, the youngest, shares the same birthday day as Tom and is eight years younger than he. Born blind, she graduated Suma cum Laude from Westminster College, In New Wilmington, Pennsylvania, where she majored in French and Spanish. Later she added German. Since August of 1989, she has operated a home business titled Lengua-Learn Communications, where "good communications lead to good relations."

After our marriage in January, we carefully planned our first week of May honeymoon. First, we'd go south on the historical National Road (Rt. 40), then head east, visiting the Assateague Island National Seashore in Virginia, and stay there for two or three days. Next, we'd head west, stop at Colonial Williamsburg for a few days, and then take Skyline Drive (which runs on a chain of the Appalachian Mountains) northward towards home.

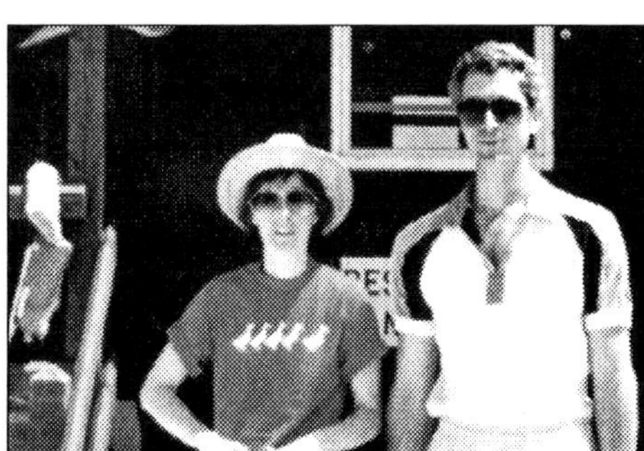
Tom and I at Chincoteague in 1987

Assateague was sunny and warm that spring, and we crammed every sunlit moment we were there, with bird watching, beach combing and bicycling along the sanctuary's trails. It was odd, but when I first saw the Assateague Island lighthouse from the car, I saw "two" lighthouses. At the beach I had a problem focusing my eyes. I blamed it on a contact lenses mix-up. (Eye problems can be a common indicator of MS.)

For a number of years, thereafter, Tom and I always held the first week of May, for our vacation, and headed down to Assateague, staying in the small town of Chincoteague. We loved the idea that we could walk to all the shops and restaurants, or bicycle while we bird watched and enjoyed nature.

In September, the same year we married, Tom's parents purchased a time-share. We met them, and his brother, Jay, down in New Bern, North Carolina for a week in October. Driving down—it was hurricane season—we ran into heavy rain and high water, surging over the Chesapeake Bay Bridge.

By the time we got to New Bern, it was dark and water was swelling over the town's only bridge. Other vehicles were flooding but our 4X4 CJ-5 made it over the bridge.

Even though Tom's dad passed away in 1982, his mother kept the time-share. Tom and I, with Jay's family, often went with her on vacation, wherever she decided to take it. Thereafter, we had two lovely vacation spots to visit each year. It was a joyous flow of life in our early marriage and over the next few years.

I'd always wanted Tom to see the rockshelter, so we took a drive there one pretty afternoon. I enthusiastically chatted the closer we got to the site. When we arrived at the foot of the shelter, I looked up and saw people at the site.

We found that Phil and a small crew from Pitt was there that day. The site had been kept dormant, and no excavating had been going on for awhile. The site lay-in-wait until future knowledge and techniques of archaeology could present data in a new light, in the exciting search for the first Americans.

Once a month, in the early years of our marriage, Tom got four days in a row off from his job with the Pittsburgh Zoo, and I had flex-hours, seven to three, at a commercial insurance company. Since Tom always had Fridays off, and I quit at three, he'd pick me up and we'd head out to his mom's in Washington County. We would meet her, Carla and Jay's family for dinner. Or, Tom and I would eat out at a local restaurant back home and then grocery shop afterwards.

On lazy, hot summer days, or colorful fall days, we'd go hiking, or fishing along the Allegheny River, north of Pittsburgh. Either, before or after our hike, we'd stop at a nearby pancake house, for a stack of blueberry pancakes, dripping with blueberry syrup.

On a day that we went Allegheny River fishing, a boat had just went by, raising the water level onto the rock where I stood. Not thinking, I took a step and gracefully slid into the river. We had planned to stop at an antique car show, and then go to a rodeo later that night. We never went to either. I was cold, soggy and wet on the ride home. Now we always carry a change of clothes in the car.

Tom and I would eventually buy bicycles from his brother, Jay, when he opened Hike'n Bike in 1989. We tried them out before we purchased them, on one of the Rails to Trails bike paths that ran alongside his shop.

I was very picky when I chose my bike from Jay, and I made it clear that I wanted a smaller wheel radius, and a low seat, like the bikes at the shore. Low enough that I could sit with my feet flat on the ground. But Tom and Jay insisted I wouldn't have enough leg stride to petal the bike properly, and that I would wear myself out quicker. They won out.

Very early in our marriage, Tom and I still believed that my pee problems were inherited. And my bulk laxative did just fine for now. I was able to adjust to the irritating, annoying bladder problems that I was experiencing—to work and lead a fairly normal life, even though I was habitually up several times a night to go to the bathroom. Though, having to pee could be a definite shouting emergency on car trips.

Slowly, the "joyful flow of life" began to backup.

7

Elusive fatigue plagued me off and on from the early '80s. I blamed it on my job—perhaps I was working overtime too much. Big projects around the house were left unfinished. I readily tired on short walks, and I kept twisting my ankles on that new pebble road along the Allegheny River—I blamed it on the clunky boots I wore.

Whirling around on a county fair ride, I grew dizzy and almost threw up. I never had this happen to me before on an amusement ride. I had another dizzy spell at home, where I lost my balance and fell on the kitchen floor. A hospital emergency doctor told me it was the flu.

In the meantime, I began researching the medical books, and I kept reading in the newspapers and magazines about that new syndrome, Chronic Fatigue. Could I possibly have it? I didn't think so, because they never mentioned the bladder problems, that now had me routinely going to an urologist.

"Can't my constant bladder infections indicate something else besides an 'overactive bladder?'" I kept asking the specialist.

He labeled my bladder: spastic or neurogenic. Because kidney ailments ran in my maternal family, I was given an Intravenous Pyelogram or IVP X-ray on my kidneys. Nothing was found.

Then one day, I was researching Tom's Merck Manual when I came upon a horrible disease called multiple sclerosis. It certainly seemed to fit my recent episodes of exhaustion, weakness and spastic bladder, and even the vertigo and numbness that I had experienced way back in college.

Reading that medical section over and over again, especially the part about extreme cases of dementia was the ultimate blow to me. It threw me back to that 3rd grade memory where a teacher called me "stupid." Losing one's mind seems so final, because it infers that your fragile soul has taken a hike.

By 1981, my nine-month job with ISO was over. The Pittsburgh office was to close due to downsizing. I started working for the company called FAIR Plan (Fair Access to Insurance Rates) in downtown Pittsburgh. With my habit of peeing, one female co-worker there gave me the nickname "Betsy Wetsy." I was still working on the bowel department by using bulk laxatives.

Then, one day, the most embarrassing event happened to me at work. I went out to pick up lunch from a delicatessen where, without warning, it hit. There I stood with a frantic look on my face, because, suddenly, my bowels had to move.

I raced out of the shop and into a five and dime store. In a panic, I hurriedly ask for the nearest ladies-room. The cashier, sensing my distress, escorted me along. There was a lunchtime crowd in the restroom, so I sat in the stall until they all had left.

I cleaned up as best I could and left to get a bus. I sat in the back and called work after I got home.

By 1985 my insurance job with FAIR Plan had also been over, due to downsizing, and I was now working for The Continental Insurance Company. In the beginning of my employment—after I'd taken the standard insurance exams—I was assured I'd be a top commercial insurance rater. But then, over the course of my five-year employment with them, I unknowingly began slipping in my responsibilities. My last job review, just before my diagnosis, had been poor.

My supervisor said, "I don't know what's wrong with you. Maybe it's your allergies."

Finally, in the summer of 1988, an internist highly suspected I had MS. While I sat on his examining table—I tried to remain calm—I spouted off my symptoms without giving away my self-diagnosis. I didn't say a word about my suspicions because I was curious to hear what this physician would say.

He examined my reflexes, looked in my eyes, and watched my gait and balance.

"What inkling or feeling do you have about these strange symptoms?" he asked after the examination.

"MS," I glumly said.

He thought so too.

Tom and I couldn't sleep that night and we cried together. But the one test the internist would give me—it measured the time it took my visual impulses to go from my eye to my brain—proved a disclaimer. Our ordinary lives went on.

Over the next months, we would go back and forth from relief to worry. Tom and I both knew that I should have made an appointment to see a neurologist, but we were reluctant, and we agonized over hearing a diagnosis that might profoundly alter the course of our relationship.

It was early May, of 1989, and we were back at Chincoteague, Virginia. I was able to maneuver the rental bike I was riding on (this was before Jay's bike shop) along the wide paths of the Assateague sanctuary, until we hit the corner streets of Chincoteague, where I'd become unbalanced and fall off the bike. That does it! Tom made me promise to go see a neurologist when we returned home.

I made a neurology appointment with a group of doctors located near the main Pittsburgh hospitals and universities. A MRI (Magnetic Resonance Imaging) X-ray was scheduled for me. It, along with observable symptoms, showed I had MS. It was somewhat of a relief to have it confirmed.

The neurologist phoned me at work with the results. I asked him if the disease might go into remission, or maybe never return.

"Perhaps," he replied.

"Would taking vitamins help?" I asked.

Then he said, "It can't hurt."

Multiple sclerosis is a disease of the central nervous system (CNS). It affects the nerves that comprise the brain and spinal cord. Its cause is unknown, it cannot be prevented, and neither a cure nor a safe and effective treatment has been able to "halt" its progression to date. Multiple sclerosis refers to multiple areas of patchy scarring, or plaques, that result from demyelination (destruction) of myelin. Myelin is a fatty insulation covering the nerve fibers. The general theory for the development of MS is that a genetically damaged immune system is unable to distinguish between virus proteins and the body's own myelin and produces antibodies that attack. In other words, the body becomes allergic to itself, a condition known as autoimmunity.

Now, I had an explanation for my neurogenic bladder, constipation, vertigo, fatigue, numbness and double vision (diplopia). Optic neuritis or inflammation of the eye is the most common vision problem for MS'ers. The protective myelin surrounding the nerve fibers is damaged in optic neuritis. It can cause blurred vision, blind spots and pain.

According to the experts, four types represent the disease: "relapsing-remitting, primary-progressive, secondary-progressive and progressive-relapsing." The latter three forms generally fall under the category of chronic-progressive MS. (At the time I was diagnosed these confusing classifications weren't yet named.)

When I had my MRI X-ray, in June of 89, it was fairly recent in its application to MS. Previously, clinical evidence of disturbing central nervous system (CNS) lesions, were found through spinal taps. That, along with a history of remissions and exacerbations, was the main tool for diagnosis.

To beat down the symptoms I was put on a course of oral steroids.

The steroids the neurologist prescribed for me caused mental confusion, which made my work performance look bad. So instead of a top-notch Continental rater or a "crack rater," I became a "crackpot rater" while on caffeine coffee and steroids. It wasn't long after my diagnosis that I told my supervisor of my MS condition, and she gave me a lighter workload.

I began slipping at work. I fell twice, once coming into the building, and once getting onto a fourth floor elevator. Another time, I was standing by a computer when my ankle gave away, causing me to almost fall. I began a better habit then falling, when I started taking the steps rather than the elevator. I was walking around the office a lot, too. I didn't want to stop moving for fear the MS would grab me.

The steroids wore off and I went back to the doctor complaining about horrendous fatigue. The anti-viral drug Amantadine was prescribed. It was incredible how effective it was, and soon I was feeling like my old self.

By June of '89, I was emotionally prepared to accept the

MS results. No, I didn't run around screaming and crying that my life was over. Nor, did I crawl into bed and pull the covers over my head, determined to be depressed for days on end. Always an oversensitive little wimp, this new toughness was different. Where did this staunchness come from? Since I saw Mom handle my father's death so well, I looked to my mother's family.

"Annie Get Your Gun"

8

Standing atop the Laurel Mountains, in the spring of 1770 or there about, you might catch a glimpse of tethered oxen, slowly winding their way around the Allegheny Mountains in southwestern Pennsylvania, perhaps by way of the Cumberland Gap, and Braddock's Road.

The fifteen or twenty families arrived some time in the spring, it is thought. A few of these settlers were Edward Harnett, John McNair, William Rush and his son, Jacob, along with Nathaniel Skinner and his son, Ruben. All my maternal great grandfathers, they settled in the Turkeyfoot region of Somerset County, Pennsylvania.

I used to joke to my Aunt Patti that my MS was a result of all the inbreeding our ancestors did. (This was before I learned of a paternal cousin's MS.)

I came to an interesting revelation after I read a cousin's rendition of my great grandmother, Annie Harned, (Figure 1), late of Somerset County. To me she was just a lovely, little old lady who told neat family stories, but my cousin Bobby Robinson sighted a different picture.

Grandma Beal was an incredibly strong woman, both physically and mentally. Although of small stature she worked beside her husband (if he was away she did it all) farming and milking, by hand, a dozen or more dairy cows every morning as well as all the other chores that went with farm life. She was one tough lady.

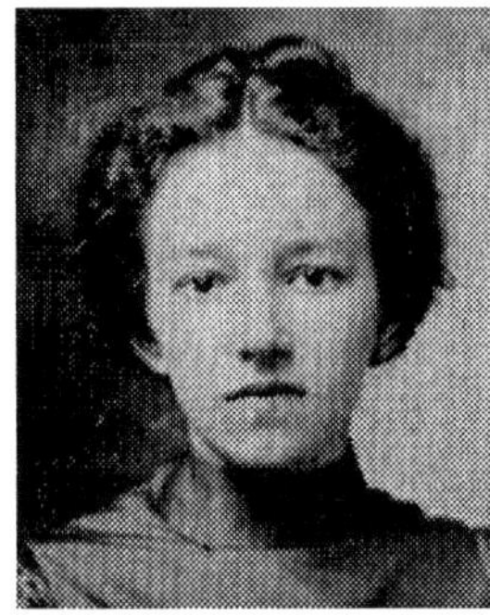

Figure 1 - Annie Harned, age 17 (1881-1978) (Courtesy RJ Robinson)

Annie worked very hard for everything she got. When anyone tried to steal her chickens, and if her husband was away at his job, she would empty her .32 caliber Smith and Wesson revolver into the direction of the chicken coop from her bedroom window. Her chickens were not bothered very much, especially one night when she put all five rounds into the door of the chicken coop and a car was heard speeding away from the vicinity. Even at 96 years of age she was still quite capable and kept up with world and local news.

I began to realize that "shades of Annie" were in me. The following job loosing incident happened in 1980, back when I was working at the soon to be closed ISO.

When the "beheading" New York City man arrived, I went in for my meeting with him in the manager's office. Feeling I didn't have anything to lose, and before he could begin his tirade, I asked, "So, will I be here the same time next year?"

"No," he said.

I went back to my desk and cried.

A few days later—I was sitting in for the receptionist—

when a New York boss telephoned and asked to speak to the manager. I almost devilishly said, "I'm sorry, he's no longer with us," but bit my tongue.

This next story was later, when I worked for The Continental Insurance Company. It would be my last job. Just like ISO and FAIR Plan, this Pittsburgh office, too, was preparing to close. Because my commercial rating ability had been slipping, I wasn't given a written recommendation to the new office—soon to be opened in York, Pennsylvania.

I heard about my "absent recommendation" when the main office sent a personnel manager to the Pittsburgh branch—for a private meeting with each of us—to discuss our future with the company.

Two other girls and I were not called. Naturally, by day's end, the entire building knew that we hadn't made the cut. How humiliating.

The next morning, I formulated an adamant, clear speech and went into the office manager, and without anger, said something like: "The handling of this situation was totally unprofessional. It was tacky, tasteless and demeaning."

They vowed to be more tackful in their office methods.

With that ill manner of treatment out of the way, another situation soon cropped up surrounding the same issue. We were sitting at our computer workstations one morning, talking about the office closing, when a female employee said, "You know, anyone without a letter of recommendation won't receive a severance pay. It's in our new handbook."

I stood up and said, "What?! We were told that anyone who stayed until closing would get a severance pay." (Of course I hadn't read the handbook.)

Back into the manager's office I went, and asked if this information were true. He immediately turned and made a call to the main office, and promptly discovered he'd told us the wrong thing. Because of the official mistake, those two other girls and myself received our severance pay.

While I was an employee with this company, I tried intermittent self-catheration every morning and evening. (Up until today, I've used every prescription drug available to control my bladder spasms.) I quit when I gave myself an infection while on a vacation in Chincoteague. Another infection resulted after a urology visit. The invasive, infection-causing practice is so uncomfortable, too. It may make it easier for the hospitals and nursing homes, but it "irritates me."

After I was given the prognosis of MS and a few months before my Continental office closing, God gave me something else to test my strength.

9

I was attending a watercolor class in the fall of 1989 when I first heard the news. Back in her hometown of Connellsville, sixty miles southeast of Pittsburgh, my mother was out raking leaves. Afterwards, she began having pelvic and back pain, and she thought that perhaps another kidney stone was on the move.

She went to her doctor on September 27th, for an examination and a pelvic sonogram. It went well so she said. She didn't give me the full story, because I know now that, her right kidney showed a 4-5mm calcification, after she had a renal sonogram, on October 8th. The physician referred her for further evaluation.

One night, when I returned home from art class, Tom gave me the startling news. Mom's sister, Patti, had telephoned from Silver Spring, Maryland, and said that my mom was in the Mt. Pleasant Hospital, and that she had been admitted on November 8th for medical tests.

I was taken aback because Mom had always been healthy and youthful. Strangers used to think we were sisters. My high school friends always thought she was cool, especially in her mini skirt (although, not too mini) and white go-go boots.

So that song about the widowed wife...who wore her mini–skirt into the room ("Harper Valley PTA") became an instant favorite, after she had given a speech, at our local high school PTA.

On the other hand, "Lady Madonna" wasn't, and she made it perfectly clear while I was playing it one day. She wasn't really a floozy, teaching Sunday school and volunteering in the church nursery.

I rushed home to Connellsville; the weekend mom was to have a liver biopsy. Patti drove up from Silver Spring.

When we got there, the hospital let us take her out to lunch. She seemed tired.

Today, now, I sit reading her medical records. On November 9th I see she had an enhanced CT Scan which revealed "evidence of wide spread metastatic disease involving the left and right lobes of the liver."

So, an attempt was made, on Nov. 11th, to do a bedside needle biopsy. Only mildly successful, it came back normal. The doctors were suspicious and setup another biopsy. On the 14th a surgeon did an open liver biopsy. A consultation with an oncologist that day reveals, "Patient's liver functions are grossly abnormal."

When Aunt Patti and I arrived at the hospital later that morning, Mom was upset, because the doctors had already done the painful liver biopsy before we got there. Of the abnormal liver Mom said nothing. Because she insisted the spots were calcium deposits, we didn't bother to read her medical chart.

I was back at work in Pittsburgh, and Patti was in the hospital with Mom, when the results of the biopsy were in. I was nervous all morning. Then the phone call came. I took it in a conference room. Patti was in Mom's hospital room and talked to me first.

"Is it cancer?" I asked her.

"Yes," she quietly said.

Then my mom spoke to me, crying all the while.

After I hung up, I ran out of the room crying. My supervisor drove me home.

I rushed back to Connellsville.

She is the only mother I'll ever have. Born July 1929, the eldest child of John Beal and Sarah "Margaret" Havner, she was named Jean "Audrey" Beal after her Aunt Jean Beal, her dad's youngest sibling. Because they were only eight years apart, it became confusing with both "Jeans," so the family started calling her Audrey.

In December of 1935 Harry was born, followed by Patricia. To Patti, her older sister had always seemed like a mother, because she had helped care for her since birth.

In caring for her little sister, Mom gained experience in childcare, and perhaps this is one reason Mom did such a fine job in raising me. Though an only child, I wasn't coddled or spoiled. Exaggerated injuries, for which I received lectures, got me little sympathy.

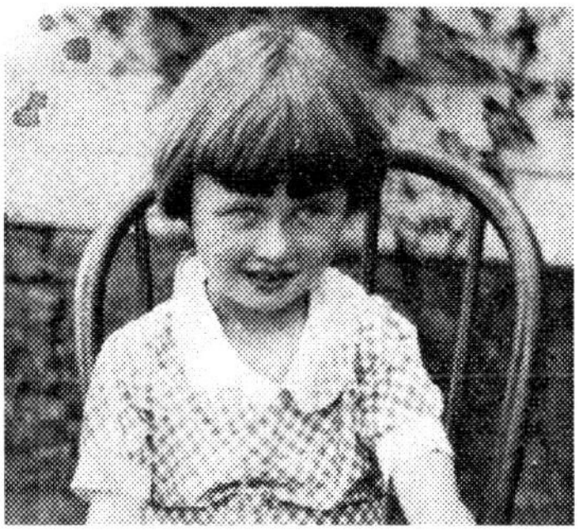

My mother, Audrey Beal

I think mother fared well in her early upbringing, in Confluence, Somerset County. She probably received much attention from her doting paternal aunts, Jean, Irma, Betty, Hazel and Rene. All the girls had manners and style.

They were a close-knit family, all getting along well together. Even Mom's good-natured Uncle Ernest "loved being around his family.... He was quick to put up the swing for visiting youngsters and always maintained the Laurel Hill Creek 'dam' for the old swimming hole," says Cousin Bobby.

My mother was very much wanted and loved.

When she was released from the hospital, the doctor told us to do everything we could to have a good time together. Patti and I tried to setup a memorable weekend.

So she didn't tire, we borrowed a wheelchair from a friend, and took her out to lunch. Then it was a little Christmas shopping, and later that day, the whole family met for dinner at a local restaurant. Afterward, we drove through a Christmas light display that always drew large crowds every year. She was exhausted by evening.

Our Thanksgiving that year was very sad indeed. Mom stayed in bed most of the day, as Patti, my cousin Kim and I prepared the meal. All around the table, Mom, my grandma Beal, Aunt Patti, my uncle Don, his mother, Cousins Jeff and Kim, and I sat. Was she sorrowful for the happy, pleasant Thanksgivings of our past? If she was, she didn't share her thoughts.

After Thanksgiving, Patti stayed awhile with Mom. I returned to work at Continental until Christmas, when I would take a leave of absence.

After Patti returned home to Maryland, mom's left leg began swelling. And she had a fever and chills. When a friend and neighbor saw her, she immediately phoned the hospital. She finally persuaded Mom to go to the emergency room, and she drove her to the hospital.

An examination found "acute thrombophlebitis." The health center put her on Coumadin and discharged her 12/8. For the first time these words appear in the discharge summary,

"Unknown malignancy–probably GI."

I'm not exactly sure when her oncologist began to speak the word "terminal" but I was on the kitchen phone at my house when I asked him, "How long?"

"Three months at the most," he replied.

Perhaps she was too gravely ill to make decisions for her care, but Mom ultimately put the decision-making on her family. We tried to encourage her to come to Pittsburgh for better treatment. Since she was terminal, what was the point in all these tiring tests and x-rays? Would stopping them mean resignation?

We never got to take her on that trip to Florida because she was so ill.

How was my MS with all this emotional stress? Walking the long hospital halls, became an excruciating effort, like I'd been mining coal. Forever! If you don't put up a constant fight, it can grab you, and ruin your chance for a normal life with cherished loved ones. I felt awful when it was so emotionally important to me to relish my mother's last days.

It was around Christmas time and I was on my leave-of-absence from work, staying again with Mom at her house. Walking in the local grocery store, I leaned on the cart for support. Back from shopping, I pulled into the garage, and suddenly my bowels had to move. I rushed into the bathroom, off the guestroom, but couldn't get my clothes undone in time.

Mom's illness took its emotional toll on Tom, too. It wasn't always apparent to me, since I was in Connellsville and he was in Pittsburgh. Tom's stress and frustration really manifested itself while he was out running errands back home.

A fellow had hit the right front fender of our car and kept on going. In anger, Tom took off after him. Catching up with him at the corner of Penn and Negley, Tom jumped out of the car and tried to rip the guy's license plate off. A man at a nearby bus stop cheered him on.

On his off days, Tom would make the one and a half-hour drive to see us. He thought a great deal of my mother and would sit in bed with her, and put his arm around her and talk.

On January 8, 1990, she was re-admitted to the hospital. Loosing weight and suffering with anemia, she was treated with a transfusion. The abnormal liver really became apparent when she began to vomit bile. As I sat holding her hand, she admired my ring. I told her I was very proud of her. Funny how we change these awful moments into something more.

The last time Mom was admitted to the health center, on February 9th, she showed signs of acute gastroenteritis, with sharp pain and a drop in her hemoglobin. Because of her poor appetite, malnutrition and nausea, a triple subclavian line was put in place for feeding. With GI bleeding now apparent, she became severely weak. Chemotherapy was withheld.

I'm glad I never read the summaries or her reports back then. It would have been too painful. I've collected disjointed remnants of memories. I recall the red socks with hearts I bought her for St. Valentine's Day. When I put them on her it put a grin on her face. I brought flowers too. She was always getting flowers.

Around February 21st, it came time for her to be discharged. I had to decide what to do next. If Mom went home with the line, I'd have to care for and perhaps utilize the ports. Not comfortable or confident, especially with MS clumsiness, I was afraid to do so. Then there was the possibility of kidney dialysis being the next step. So I regretfully decided she should enter the nursing home down the road from the health center.

I found out just how upset she was in the home, after friends informed me of her crying. She stayed only one week, when I told the staff to remove the line. She was coming home—no more tubes and no dialysis.

There were warm, sunny days that March, and I encouraged her to come out on the sun porch with me. She came out with my help for a few minutes, and then went back to bed.

The oncologist prescribed oral morphine for her pain. I began taking her to radiation. I began slurring my words.

Cooking healthy meals, I tried to entice her. I made the homemade bean soup she wanted, but she got sick afterwards. It would be her last meal.

The night of March 22, she called to me while I slept down in the basement bedroom. I went up to see to her and then went back to bed. I was mentally, emotionally and physically exhausted. I wish I'd crawled into bed with her like Tom did.

I was up that morning and I could tell she was slipping into a coma. Tom soon came and was concerned about her comfort level. He wanted to give her a morphine injection, but it was unauthorized. Instead, it was administered via a suppository.

I tried to phone Aunt Patti, and since there was no answer, I thought perhaps she was on her way. She arrived, and soon we were all by her bedside, including Cousin Virginia and the minister.

By 3:00 Patti and I were holding her hands, sobbing. Mom fought and struggled when she heard grandma crying in the next room. I wiped her face, with a wet facecloth, and she became calmer. I ask her if that felt good and she nodded yes. By 3:30 she was gone.

10

Once in a while that spring, I'd sit gazing out a window or an open door, pensive and wistful and full of sorrow, while watching the sun move across the floor. It was during one of these moments that I started reflecting on previous family funerals that I had witnessed.

I came to the death of my maternal great-grandpa, Franklin Havner, and I was sure I'd witnessed his funeral at a very young age. Mother said I was two years old, too young to recall that event. Had she been mistaken about my age perhaps?

It came to me to dig into my old genealogy charts from the 70's and look at death dates. Yes, indeed, I discovered I wasn't two, but three and a half years old—old enough for it to have left its mark.

Could genealogy reveal any further mysteries of my family? I was curious to learn more. So I began picking up where I'd left off in my genealogy, years earlier.

To start, I looked up my cousin Bobby (I discovered he'd also been working on our tree) whom I hadn't seen or talked to in 20 years, and together we delved into the past.

After his mom had passed away, Bobby found a lamenting and yearning letter in his mom's belongings, harking back to another cousin's long ago family. This letter expresses my longing behavior after my mom passed away.

Camp on or near the Potomac in Maryland. Sept. - 1862

Dear Unkle, Aunt, & Relations

I have not heard of you but as you are near & dear to me I thought I would spend my leasur moments in penning a few lines to you. you are many miles away from me, mountains & valleys intervene. You all are sitting around (least I hope so) at home surrounded with all the dainties and comforts of life whilst I am here being a soldier surrounded with many persons engaged in the same cause of crushing out a rebellion that is unjust to all.

I have been over some parts of the late battlefields known as the South Mountain & Sharpsburg Battle fields. Some of the most Horrible sights man could see I have seen but I stood it very well as it was nothing more than I expected to see.

I have seen persons with their legs torn nearly off. one man shot in the brest torn at least half into and indeed many in all forms among or surrounded with these sights & more dead. Horses lying around sending up some of the most fragrant of smells.

I have cooked and eaten my dinner not with as much relish as I have partook of some meals but then there are things that a soldier must not mind for if I live I expect to see some sights just as hard if not harder than these. I do wish you could be here or in the Battlefield to see the horrors of war. You can form ideas but nothing compares with reality.

We were marched with all speed to this place. One week we were on the march. Some nights we marched all night. Such is soldiering with 60 rounds of cartridge in the box gun knapsacks on our sholdiers all, making a right good load. Also our rations

& canteens full of water but a soldiers life is a soldiers life.

Hard it is to stand up to the hardships of it too yet I hope that I will get through safe. We are here now but don't know how long we will remain. The troops say they never fought harder than they did here. They say the rebels contested the field hard giving way inch by inch...it was heavy as easy.

I wish I was at your house to have a good meal over good sweet milk and fresh butter. Oh how I would enjoy it but if I live to get back I will call on you for all these things knowing that if I do so I shall receive. There are many pleasures here to share & time passes swiftly away yet none do I enjoy as much as the drill when I am well yet I am content with my lot.

Let it be as it will sick or well I know that I shall endeavor to live in a way that will be pleasing in the sight of God. He can and will protect those that put their trust in Him. As He led the children of Israel through dangers so will He or at least He has promised to guide and protect those that put their trust in Him.

May we all live so that when death overtakes us let it be in what way it will. May it be sweet to die but through or under His protection I hope to greet you again after the many dangers that threaten us at all times are o'er and passed.

May we all press onward and upward to the high calling which is through Christ the living head from whence all good cometh is my prayer but I must close wishing you all will accept my best wishes for your comfort & happiness one & all and if I live to get back may we meet as Christians ought to meet to part no more and may the rebellion be tramped out neler to rise again.

Now if I live to get back you must kill me a chicken, have some good sweet milk, some good fresh butter & bread and then I can eat, oh with an apetite that will astonish you if – I never had such an apetite as I had before I got sick.

Nothing more but remain your loving Nephew until death
Judson S. Hartzell

(Special Note - Judson S. Hartzel, Sgt., War of the Rebellion, Co. E, 133rd Regiment was mustered in August 14,1862 and out May 26, 1863 per records at the Somerset Historical Society. Discovered & read with great pleasure by Robert James Robinson June 30, 1993.)

11

In May of 1990, Tom and I took the bikes we got from Jay's shop to Assateague, for some relaxation and bird watching. I was able to glide with ease along the straight, wide and level sanctuary trails, even though I had balance problems. Whenever I went to stop, Tom would steady the bike for me, so it wouldn't pull me over. It was time to repair my health and heal my soul.

But the MS would not retreat, and I returned home, in June, to a course of oral steroids, with poor results. It was my intention to regroup and go back to work. Because of my flair up, and with no apparent remission in sight, Tom and I decided I should apply for a Social Security disability.

Tom and I started thinking about a dog to keep me company and went to see a litter of Dalmatian puppies. Dalmatians are such whimsical, charming creatures, and we fell in love with the puppies soon after they were born. Darling Abbey fit right in when we brought her home.

Meanwhile, Social Security turned me down. I resubmitted. And for the second time I was rejected. Rather then reapply, I contacted a disability attorney.

I told my story straightforward, into a microphone, while Judge Ira Fundy sat upon his platform. He asked the questions—I gave the answers.

It was certainly a little odd, though, that old apartment roommate, the one who pulled "Apartment Edie" off me, took down my initial interview with the attorney.

The Social Security disability finally came through while Tom and I were in the Smokey Mountains of North Carolina, with his mom and sister, Carla. Friends of ours, Vince and Cathy, and their two dogs, stayed at our place to Abbey sit. Cathy read me the conformation letter over the phone.

It was on this trip that I suffered a bazaar allergic incident, over a few lousy crumbs from a peanut butter cookie. They were on the piece of sugar cookie that I made sure to brush off before I attempted to eat it. I didn't think a few crumbs would matter, but afterwards, for caution, I took an antihistamine.

Then Tom and I went out to get gas for the car when I suddenly started getting sick. We rushed back. In the bath I began throwing up, so Tom administered an injection (.02cc) of Epinephrine. When that didn't help he gave me another injection.

Here we were, in the beautiful Great Smokies, miles from a decent hospital. We ended up on a long nighttime drive over a winding road to a country hospital in Linville. I was kept a couple of hours for observation.

Back home, by the fall of '90, my walking had deteriorated. At first, I was able to walk Abbey at least once around the block when we brought her home in August. After that, it went to half a block, and then to half a block with a cane. Tom and I realized I should have wheeled transportation if I was to have any outdoor fun. We decided on a rugged Triumph, a heavy-duty 3-wheeled electric scooter.

I thought I'd try another avenue in combating the MS, seeing a local homeopathic doctor in the spring of 1991. Eight vials of blood were drawn and sent to an antibody lab in California where results showed a presence of an activated cellular immune system in the positive range. Part of the holistic treatment included allergy injections which I administered myself.

You can see, from the below, an immune system in overkill.

	MY RESULTS	RANGE
%TA1 POSITIVE CELLS	30.00	0.00 to 8.00%
TA1 POSITIVE CELLS	630.00	0.00 to 256.00
INTERLEUKIN 1 GENERATION	15.00	2.70 to 7.60 Ng/ml
MYELIN AUTOANTIBODIES (IgG)	negative	negative

In 1991, Tom rode the 150-mile MS Bike Tour, a two-day, one-way trip from Pittsburgh, north to Erie. He stayed overnight in a noisy college dorm. The MS Tour provided buses for the trip back to Pittsburgh. His brother, Jay, raised over $2,000 from his heavy equipment customers. Tom loved the scenic vantage point the bicycle gave him on the road to Erie.

By '92 I no longer drove because my lower legs were going numb, at intervals, and my right foot began dropping—all of which could slow my reaction time. To combat the "foot drop" I started wearing a small plastic "L" shaped brace. It was given to me by a physical therapist whom freely stop at my house a few times to give me exercise advice. I lightly exercised with ankle weights, too.

When walking and lifting my feet became more difficult, I was fitted for leg braces made at a local rehab center. But I didn't like them, because they threw out my hips and restricted my walking to an ungainly stride.

Another therapy expert eventually told me I hadn't been fitted right. By this time, though, I didn't want the damn things. The local rehab center said I should return and be refitted. I never did go back.

Besides using a scooter I began using a walker. Tom purchased a four-wheeled walker, with handbrakes and a seat, for me to use while walking around in the house. It gave me the steadiness and support I needed.

For muscle strength and exercise I jumped into and welcomed the weightless freedom of swimming. So not to overdo the independent swim, I limited my stay in the rehab pool to 20 minutes. I went twice a week and usually went with friends Vince and Cathy.

One day after showering, I clearly noticed an energy jolt while I stood combing my hair in the locker room mirror. The bright-eyed view I saw in the mirror was momentarily sharp, reflecting a shining countenance, and for a moment I felt exuberantly revived.

Endorphins at work.

I signed up for the same swim-class three or four times, but eventually, I had to drop out each time. When I had a physical therapist begin to work with me in the pool, my left leg started locking and going ridged.

Then the effects of swimming began to set-off involuntary muscle reflexes when I tried to sleep at night. The action went from my ankles into my big toes. The medical term for this maddening toe movement is: "Babinski's sign." Tylenol halted my ankle and toe action.

For alternative punches, I was up to a little meditating and gentle yoga. The gentle stretching of yoga kept my muscles flexible and helped my spasms.

I also explored hypnotism. Members of a local group were investigating the affects it had on illness. They had been invited to my house one evening when I was having an MS meeting. However, there would be no hypnotic results for me that first gathering, or for one of my houseguests, who fell asleep, snoring.

During a more intimate gathering, though, I felt comfortable enough to slip into a guided meditation. When I awoke, I almost burst out laughing. Because I felt so silly, I kept quiet and didn't say anything. For days afterward I was beaming at a brighter world. Yes, even grocery store items were happy.

In another home encounter, it was just hypnotist Paul and I, and since I liked his technique, he readily hypnotized me. During this meeting with him I urgently had to pee. Returning to the couch he told me to count backwards from 10. I heard my voice: 10, 9, 8, 7—the 7 spoken barely above a whisper and I was under a spell again.

Then one day I got an unexpected morning phone call. It was my cousin, Lois, who I hadn't spoken to or seen since we were kids. Four years younger than me, she and I are cousins on dad's side of the family. With real concern she began describing MS like symptoms. She was a nurse, who had dealt with MS patients before, so she was wise to its manifestations. One of her early doctors wouldn't commit himself, but she was later diagnosed. Now, we especially keep in touch.

12

It was in February of 1993 that I first noticed a slight lump, high up, on the right side of my chest-wall. The year before, at age 39, I had had my first mammogram. I chose to have it done at an earlier age because of my mother's colon cancer. Anyway, breast cancer didn't run in my mother's family. I hurried in to the breast center for a mammogram. I showed them the visible lump and they did a painful biopsy right after the mammogram.

Before the results were back, a rush appointment was made to see Pittsburgh breast surgeon, Dr. Matthew Walters. After his exam, he swung a heavy burden, like an immense wrecking ball rushing towards me.

It was revelations of breast cancer. My thoughts were a blank, and I shut down, except for thinking of home. I didn't want to ponder the thought of cancer, until I was back in the nest, where I could think quietly and seek emotional solace with Tom.

After a couple of worried, nervous days for Tom and I, the lab results indicated infiltrating ductal carcinoma (IDC). After that, things moved ahead very quickly. I was just glad that I didn't have to fully face my emotions yet.

Janet, my sister-in-law, saw me through all the pre-op at the Magee-Women's Hospital. To the chest x-ray, blood work and bone scan, we took my wheeled walker (which I sat on while she pushed me). We got stares, but we laughed anyway.

The surgery date was set. A right breast lumpectomy was readily preformed and a sampling of my lymph nodes were removed. When I awoke, I knew right away that it was definitely cancer. I couldn't wait to see Tom.

After surgery, Dr. Walters spoke in private to Tom and his mom, telling them that my lymph nodes thankfully showed no sign of cancer, but that the final biopsy indicated an estrogen-receptor status. He also told them that I was an emotionally strong person.

Later that morning, he came into my hospital room singing the Beatle's song "Michele."

"You are my most chipper patient," he said. "It's up to you, would you like to go home later today or stay the night?"

I opted to stay overnight.

By evening Tom's brother, Jay, and his wife Janet, came into my hospital room carrying flowers. Uncomfortable, they didn't know what to say at first; so, I said, "I thought I was going to give birth to the 'Alien.'"

I came home from the hospital with a drain tube in my right side, right under my armpit, to collect any fluid that might build up. Every morning (before he left for work) and evening, Tom routinely emptied the plastic bulb, that the tube was attached to at the other end. We had to measure and record the residual a few times a day. Its level was supposed to go down, but in my case it always remained too full to prompt the removal of the tube, any time soon.

Besides fussing with the drain tube I was diligently doing arm-stretching exercises, so scar tissue wouldn't permanently constrict my range of motion.

After two weeks, or so, the oncology office removed my drain tube per chance of infection. Janet and I had more fun with my walker, running back and forth to my surgeon's office to have it aspirated, because of fluid buildup.

Since the carcinoma was positive for estrogen, with a greater chance of reoccurrence, I decided to take six months of chemotherapy, besides six weeks of radiation. The chemotherapy was a combination of three common anticancer drugs. They are: Cyclophosphamide or Cytoxan, Methotrexate and Fluorouracil (CMF).

A five-year hormonal treatment with Nolvadex (generic name Tamoxifen) was also on the list. This medicine would block the path of the hormone estrogen in my body.

The sun burned hot, it burned my eyes
Burned so hot I thought I died
Thought I died and gone to hell...
I saw the water from a deeper well.
(Dave Olney, Daniel Lanois, Emmylou Harris)

13

It was the first week of April—I had just completed the first treatment of my second month of chemotherapy—and I had developed what I thought was a stubborn sinus headache. When the severe headache continued—and after long napping, with MS like symptoms—my oncology office advised I should call my neurologist.

On April 10th, the Saturday before Easter, the neurological problems escalated. Getting ready for bed my left side suddenly grew weak and I lost control of my bladder. I went right to bed.

Over night the pain in my right upper temple became excruciating. It got so bad I could hardly hold my head up to look at the clock. I was too traumatized and too crushed to think straight.

In the morning my headache seemed much better; so, I got dressed. Using my wheeled walker I went into the kitchen to get breakfast. I went right for the fridge and opened the door. I stood there a moment, then shut the door. I did this three or four times in a row. Next, I went to the sink, filling a glass with water over and over. I knew what I was doing was wrong, but I couldn't stop.

I began to realize something was dreadfully wrong. Tom had to work that Easter and he'd already left. Very frightened, I immediately phoned him at the zoo.

That Easter Sunday, on the 11th, Tom and his mom took me to the emergency room at the St. Francis Medical Center, where they immediately gave me a CT scan. Afterwards, when an emergency room physician stepped into the small alcove where I lay, he told Tom and his mom to step out for a moment. I could tell by the frown and concern on his face that, whatever it was, it wasn't good.

Then he said, "There is a spot on your scan. I don't know what it is. It could be a tumor."

The scan showed a mass in the right frontal region of my head. Later, the doctors would add, with surrounding hemorrhage and edema.

I was crying when Tom and his mom stepped back in to comfort me.

Interns came in and feverishly questioned me. I gave them my old home address.

In intensive care overnight, there was concern I might have a seizure, so the anti-convulsing drug Dilantin was prescribed and I was put on a monitor.

All night along, the head of ICU ran around on the linoleum floor with wooden clogs on. I would have liked to have taken one and thrown it at him.

By early morning residents—with interns in tow—were going around reviewing the medical stories of each patient. When they finished with me and moved on, one of the residents stayed behind to talk. What he told me, I don't remember, but whatever it was, it seemed profound.

I was given a MRI X-ray and assigned to a room.

Five weeks later, my discharge summary would say the following: "Initially it was thought that this mass might be a hemorrhagic metastatic brain lesion. However, follow-up scanning indicates a hemorrhagic infarct from a venous thrombosis related to superior sagittal sinus thrombosis. A coagulopathy study was done, which did not reveal any clear-cut hypercoagulable state."

It would be suspected, however, that I might have had something like that causally related either to my BC, or possibly to the chemotherapy, or Tamoxifen. (Studies show that less than 1% of women develop blood clots either in the legs or lungs while taking Tamoxifen. The percentage for clots in the brain is even lower.) My cancer drugs were withdrawn, and an IV treatment with the steroid Decadron was begun.

What a wreck I was. At mealtime, I was propped up and restrained in a chair. Nurses had to fix my meal tray so I could eat. I floundered, struggling awkwardly, with little control. I laid there for the first couple of days sleeping, unaware of my serious situation.

My body was to be especially condemned for a good long while. I was lost, stumbling around in the "journey of death" again; only, this time it wasn't any fun.

Four days after my admittance, on the 15th, I had a repeat MRI X-ray. The right frontal showed a slight decrease in the edema. Still, there was relatively extensive, persistent white matter edema.

All in all, though, they pronounced me relatively stable compared to my condition four days earlier. More MRI X-rays would follow throughout my hospital stay.

I spent 19 days, from April 11 to April 30, in the main hospital. Next came twenty murderous days down on the 2nd floor rehab under Dr. Zimmerman. Now, they were really trying to kill me.

Since Tom was at work, it was my Aunt Patti and Uncle Don who first saw me stand and take my first agonizing steps in the rehab room. Tom would later join me in rehab on his off days. He worked with the therapist and I, so he could learn my exercise routine for back home.

Five days a week, for two hours in the morning, and two hours after lunch, I held on and forced myself to keep moving in four areas of therapy: physical, occupational, mental and daily living. It seemed I would never get any rest. Because the morning physical therapy was so taxing, and required enormous energy, the patients showered every evening after dinner.

The hospital rehab gym is the "arena" where your struggle is observed, put on display. Every Friday morning all the rehab patients lined up for Dr. Zimmerman's 9:00 o'clock evaluation. He'd walk around with one arm bent and his other hand on his chin and watch. The therapists pushed my body and they pushed my mind, but it had to be done if I wanted to recover some of what I'd lost.

Just when I thought I could nap before dinner, in comes the "head hunting" psychologist. I was still mentally intact.

I tried sneaking out of two therapy classes. One was a mind game. Before it began, I started wheeling out the door behind the therapist, when I heard a voice behind me say, "Where are you going Michele?" The other was a wheelchair volleyball game. I took my anger out in the game by slamming the ball. The elderly patients recoiled in fright.

During the first few days of my hospital care, Tom's Mom, Pat, stayed at our place. I was very glad she was there, and he sure needed her support, because over the next few weeks he would become exhausted and very strained. I could see it, and the medical records say it.

That first night, when I was in the ICU, he was on the phone constantly, with calls from my family, his family, and our friends and neighbors. Over the course of my hospital stay, he didn't know how long he could handle the stress.

My neighbor, Dr. Frank Bontempo, was the razor sharp hematologist who conducted my coagulopathy studies during my stay in the hospital. Dr. Peter Ellis was appointed my St. Francis oncologist. He was cheerful and had a good bedside manner. I later learned he was a friend of Dr. Bontempo. At the helm, too, was the all-important neurologist, Dr. David Wright, along with the head of physical therapy, Dr. Zimmerman. Together they all carried me along the path of recovery.

During the day, friends and family stopped in to see me, bringing flowers and gifts. Every evening, after work, Tom was at the hospital sitting by my side. On one such night he brought me a Klondike treat. Soon we began stashing them in the visiting room fridge. While I was on steroids, eating became my favorite pastime, and each menu was looked forward to with "relish."

Roberta or Bobbie as I called her, was one of the good-hearted nurses on the rehab floor who took care of me. Singing up and down the halls, you always knew when she was coming.

One night she asked if my laxative had worked yet.

"Yeah, I said. "Last night with nurse so and so." We laughed.

I left the hospital, on May 20th, when Tom's mother brought me home. I was anxiously looking forward to this day, ever since I'd been following a hospital calendar. However, just because I left didn't mean I was off the hook. I still had six weeks of radiation to go through, and at least five weeks of out-patient PT. I left St. Francis in a rented wheelchair until mine was ready. I was never, ever, to completely escape the chair.

Our poor pup. Abbey had really missed me so. Tom's mom let her out on the back porch to greet me when we arrived. She had been howling mournfully—carrying on every night Tom came home, late, from the hospital.

After I was home, and had time to think before the radiation and PT began, I started to realize something—that my dad and I both had our hemorrhages at the age of 40, down to the same month. (I now believe age forty to be the genetic half-life of mankind.)

Dad and I also shared the middle name Quay. I was to find out that someone else shared our name. Here is a surprising little story.

A few years after my hemorrhage, I noticed that a Mary Nicklow, from Texas, had submitted a genealogy query on the Internet. I excitedly wrote to her, and made the startling discovery that her husband is Quay Nicklow, born in El Dorado, Arkansas.

At first, we thought that maybe Quay was an old family surname, but this proved wrong. The only thing we could think of was some sort of tie to a popular U.S. Senator from Texas, Matthew Stanley Quay, who had been born in Beaver County, Pennsylvania, in 1833. Many sons were named after him.

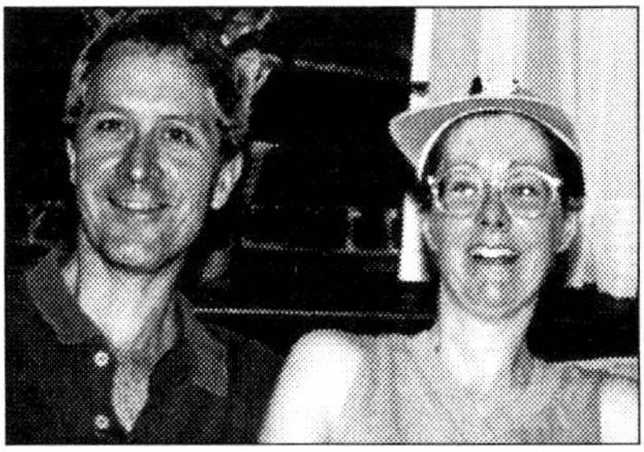
Tom and I in 1993, shortly after I got out of the hospital

Back home from the hospital, Tom had everything in place: a portable commode, a big shower bench and a ramp on to our back porch. There were new adjustments, but I was so darn happy to be home.

With Tom's mom staying on, and a few days after I'd settled in, she was in the kitchen while I was on the couch with the port-a chair next to me for easy access. I had just eaten a banana. Done using the chair, I got up holding on to only one armrest, which sent the chair off balance. It only took a second for me to tumble face first and hit the hardwood floor. When Pat pulled me up she saw I'd bitten into my now bloody lip, caused by one, now, very loose front tooth.

When Tom came through the door that night, I couldn't even look at him. Then, when I did, I cried. Treating my tooth very gingerly, I couldn't easily eat the evening meal. A specialist, recommended by a neighbor, saved my tooth.

While I was in the hospital, I decided to keep optimistic and pleasant Dr. Ellis as my permanent oncologist. In the meantime, I made one last appointment with my old one. What more could he tell me about what had happened? When I telephoned to make the appointment they were very concerned.

Before the appointed time, Tom's mom and I went and sat in the empty waiting room—and we sat.

At the front desk, I said, "It's been awhile and we are getting tired of waiting. How much longer will it be?"

"Oh, he's with another patient, and will call you soon," they said.

Again we sat.

Finally, I got disgusted, and Pat and I left.

I had missed a post-op visit with Dr. Walters, so I went to see him when I got out of the hospital, too. I was lying on the exam table, when he walked in saying, "Oh, Michele, Michele...."

He then leaned over the table and gave me a kiss on the forehead. That was sweet.

Between Tom, his mom, the help of my neighbor, Eve, and handicap transportation, I completed both PT and radiation. I never thought I'd make it through. I was very tired by 8:30 every night. After Tom helped me get ready for bed he would tuck me in. Then, he'd sit beside me while we each spoke of our day.

I liked Dr. Wright at St. Francis, and he remained my neurologist when I left. He put me on the prescription Baclofen, since Tylenol no longer helped my muscle spasms and rigidity. I'd already quit Amantadine, because it no longer worked effectively.

During one Dr. Wright office visit, he and I sat and spoke about what had happened in spring of '93.

I nonchalantly said, "Oh, I guess it wasn't too bad with all that happened."

"Oh, no, you really shouldn't be here," he emphatically said.

I was shocked.

While I slept that night three scenarios haunted my mind—each one successively more powerful.

"God Does Not Play Dice"
(Other Worlds by Physicist Paul Davies)

14

In the first dream I'm visiting a neighbor, to welcome home their new baby. Holding the baby in my arms, I notice to my horror that it has the face of a gremlin. I don't know if they're aware of this, but I don't want to let on. So I pretend there is nothing wrong. I call this dream "The Denial."

In the next, I'm riding up in a crowded elevator. We pass the 13th floor and stop on 14. I jokingly comment, "Well at least we didn't stop on 13."

When the doors open into the bright light, I immediately see we're atop the building. Suddenly, people grab my arms, and begin propelling me towards the edge. I realize they're going to throw me off the roof. This one I call "The Abyss."

In the third dream, I'm walking into a house carrying a backpack. Entering an airy kitchen, I begin taking things out of the bag, while talking to a couple of folks. I know I'm there for a reason, but just don't know why.

Walking upstairs and down a hall, I begin to have creeping, dreadful feelings the closer I get to a bathroom. The stark white bath is empty except for a clear glass, sitting on the sink. In the glass is a hypodermic needle. I pick it up. Horrified, I realize I'm here to give myself a lethal injection. I turn, run down the stairs, out the door, into the arms of my family.

I call the above dream the "The Choice." Does God give us a choice or does he say, "No, not now?"

This is where it started, with these three almighty dreams. I began pondering my mortality. I can't ignore the signs now. I'm beginning to feel that my life's journey was already written and stamped by God. The acknowledgment of the Jumonville Cross I kept buried, although I never forgot about it. It wasn't until I wrote this section of my story that I began to accept its power. Throw in the Meadowcroft Rockshelter (a symbol of "mankind") and you have quite a mix.

I have never been a religious person, but now I've started reading the Bible that I haven't opened since junior high school. It's beginning to sound like *Close Encounters*. All of a sudden, God is calling me? I never thought God would want me.

I didn't, in the least, begin to grasp His message until I started writing about what I felt were the most outstanding events of my life. Before, I was cynical—yeah, sure, like writing it all down is going to make a difference—about those, so-called, "gratitude journals."

How can you think or feel one way, one moment, and then do a turn around the next? Accepting new and different concepts in life can be a challenge, because its process exposes the vulnerability in us all. Transforming words can connote all sorts of earth-shattering episodes: transfiguration, transceiver, transmit, transcendental and trance.

Now if I live to get back,
you must kill me a chicken.
Have some good sweet milk,
some good fresh butter & bread.
And then I can eat,
oh, with an apetite, that will astonish you.
(Judson S. Hartzel)

15

With my right leg swelling, I was admitted into the St. Margaret Medical Center, a few days before the 1995 Thanksgiving Holiday. Tom and I feared another blood clot. An emergency room ultra-sound readily showed the dreaded clot. They administered a course of Heparin to thin my blood.

Over the Thanksgiving weekend I cried to my Aunt Patti on the phone. I sent Tom to his moms for his turkey dinner. He didn't feel like staying long. It was a lonely time to cry; to invoke and retreat to the happy Thanksgiving Holidays of before—another family gathering sorely missed.

I was released after four days, and took with me a different neurologist—one that was associated with St. Margaret. My new neurologist updated my MS medical record with a MRI X-ray, and she had my brain waves (electroencephalogram or EEG) tested. The electrodes attached to my head would reveal possible brain abnormalities. I never looked at the results.

A racing pulse that had been found during my admittance to the hospital revealed that my heart was beating too rapidly. Blood work confirmed I'd been slapped with hyperthyroidism or Grave's disease. Again, my body was attacking itself.

Your immune system uses antibodies (protein substances the body makes) to help protect itself against viruses, bacteria and foreign substances (antigens) that invade your body. In Grave's disease, your immune system mistakenly attacks your thyroid gland, and your skin and assail the tissue behind your eyes causing Grave's ophthalmopathy (opf-thal-mop-athy). The eyes may bulge. You may experience sensitivity to light, blurring or double vision, inflammation or decreased eye movement. Although the cause of Grave's disease is unknown, it is believed that a combination of factors including your family heredity, immune system, gender and age may attract it.

I already have a "grave disease" and I don't need another. Grave's disease is a body constantly running in overdrive. Months before, I'd become a short tempered, argumentative, cranky, cantankerous insomniac but with all my other troubles, I never gave these clues a second thought. My thyroid was slowly killed off with radio–iodine I–131 and I was put on Synthroid.

Everyday I could feel the downward destruction of the MS. Like chills, numbness surged up and down my spine at night.

Nerve endings began to hound me constantly. It was like being stabbed with endless hundreds of tiny needles. I thought I'd go absolutely crazy, spinning my wheelchair around and around in the middle of the kitchen floor. My new doctor prescribed the wonder drug Nortriptylin, and it nixed all the harassment, before it drove me completely insane.

"I always said I would make her a deed, and, don't you think, I ought to do it?" (John Brooks to Alexander Hanna)

16

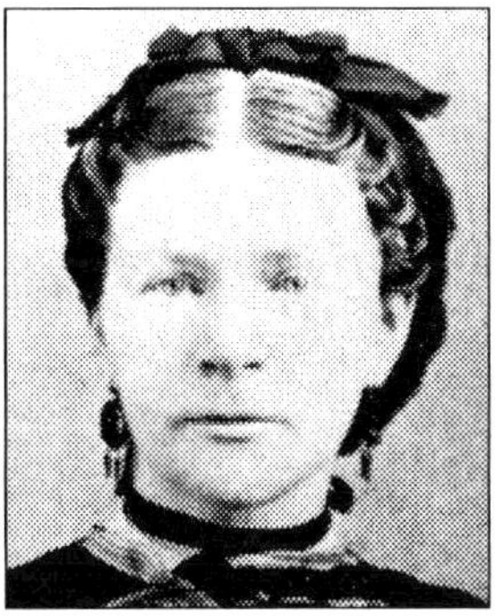

Figure 2 - Mary Ann Brook (1839-1879) (Courtesy RJ Robinson)

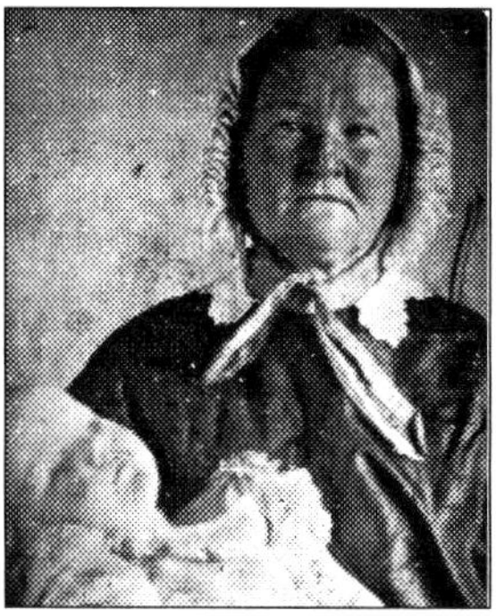

Figure 3 - Jane Hanna & grandchild (1810-1880) (Courtesy RJ Robinson)

Using the fine example of mother raising me and seeing her struggles after my father's death, coupled with my observation of other emotionally strong female family members, gives credence to my fight. Besides Mom and Great Grandma Annie Harned, I strongly identify with my 3rd great-grandmother, Mary Ann Brook (Figure 2).

I've uncovered detailed court documents that grasp an in-depth portrait of Mary Ann and her family. Like other females in my family, she gives the appearance of a woman with backbone.

In 1857, Mary Ann marries Edward Harned, but he dies in 1867, at age 32. Later, a 24-year-old Mattie Brook—Mary Ann's only surviving sibling—passes away in December of 1869. Then their father, John Brook, suddenly dies in November of 1870. Intestate, he leaves Mary Ann and her

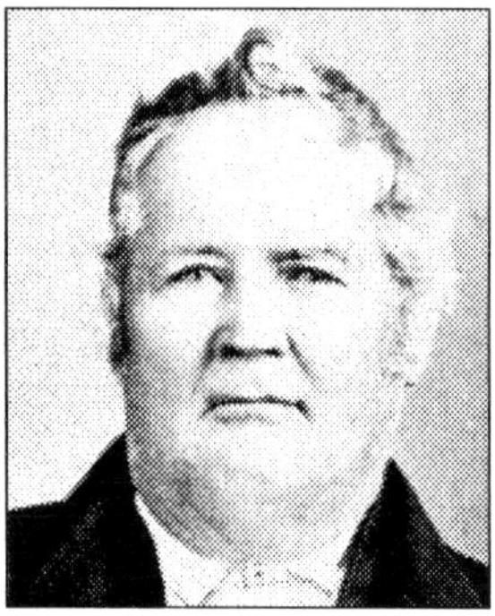
Figure 4 - William "Uncle Billy" Hanna (1805-1890) (Courtesy RJ Robinson)

mother, Jane Hanna (Figure 3), a legal mess with an estate and accounts to be settled.

A few months later, in May of 1871, Mary files a petition for a farm she says her father gave her as a "verbal gift." After lengthy testimony, on September 16th, 1871, the court grants her deed to the property. Eight days later, her 8-year-old son, Milton, dies.

If you could get an overall feel, or paint a vivid picture of an 1870'S farming community, Mary Ann's court records surely show it. I've come to know these "Turkeyfooters," of Turkeyfoot Twp., who talk to you.

Mary Ann's uncles, William and Alexander (Figures 4 and 5) Hanna were sworn as witnesses, and made their statements in behalf of Mary Ann and her farm.

WILLIAM HANNA, AFFIRMED

In the fall of 1868, 1 went with parties to Mrs. Mary A. (Brook) Harneds' to rent the farm, on which she was living. She said other parties had been there to rent, and she had requested her father to Superintend the renting & referred us to him. We then called upon him, he, said the property belonged to her and he, preferred her renting it herself and would do nothing until he would confer with her. I know that she occupied the property 10 or 12 years.

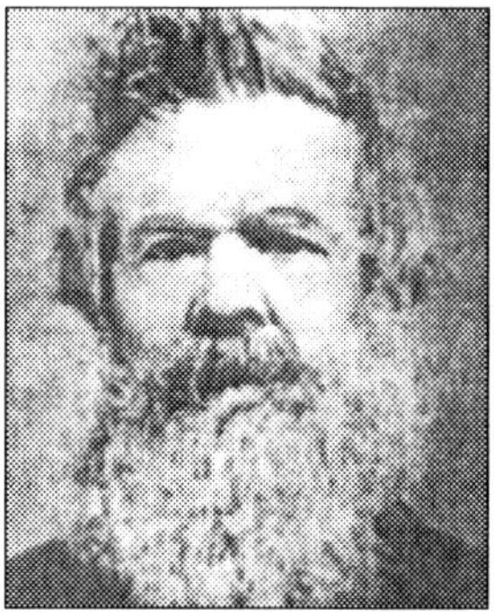
Figure 5 - Alexander Hanna (1802-1880) (Courtesy Michael Connelly)

MAJOR ALEXANDER HANNA, ESQ, SWORN.
In frequent conversations, with John E. Brook, I always understood from him that he had given the, "Brick House" place to his daughter Mary Ann in the early part of 1870. He spoke to me about writing deeds for this farm and a farm, which Edward King Harned had purchased from him. He said, "I always said I would make her a deed and don't you think, I ought to do it?" Mary Ann (Brook) Harned lived on the property about twelve years. On the first of Jan 1869, I wrote an agreement for Mary Ann, renting the farm to E.D. Yutzey. Yutzey stated that because Mrs. Harned had no deed, her right to rent might be disputed by her father and he wished her father to sanction the agreement. I then wrote an approval, for Yutzey, at the bottom of the agreement that Brooks' had signed.

Mary Ann didn't sit back and just say, "Oh well, it will all work out," leading a happenstance life. In her words: "I made improvements on the farm. Built a grain house and sugar house and repaired the dwelling house, built & repaired the fences, cultivated and improved the land."

She maps her direction and because of her efforts, she's able to hand down the farm to her descendants. I realize belatedly that to make a real significance in life you have to go the extra distance with gusto and passion.

I used to practice the old "John Brook" habit of saying "don't you think I ought to do it," and then do nothing about it. My new resource, the "Mary Ann" method of toughness, was always there, lying dormant until it was needed. Always laid-back, I now see that her method should have been applied to all I tackled in life.

After the death of her first husband, Mary Ann remarried and bore son "Willie," but Willie died a few days after his first birthday. She was already one month pregnant with another child, and so a second son was born to her on April 25, 1879.

Then possibly due to complications of childbirth, Mary passed away on May 14, 1879, at age 39. Because she died just three months shy of her 40th birthday, I feel a close link with her.

In keeping with my mother's toughness, I can remember one Sunday childhood afternoon scrabbling and scrounging around under a neighbor's front porch, in clean clothes that were to stay that way. Afterwards, I whined and complained that I wanted cleaned up, and changed into clean clothes.

"Nope," my mother said, "you made your choice. You'll just have to live with it the rest of the day."

Now that I look back, I think Mom must have let me wonder through life early, in a free roaming atmosphere of fun learning mixed with sound judgement, practicality and common sense. She let me make my own choices, because she trusted my reasoning and course of action. And when she didn't, she made it perfectly clear. You learn a more distinct path by experiencing the many consequences of your decisions.

"Breast cancer doesn't run in my family."

17

Now, it's February 23, 1998, my five-year cancer window, and I'm scheduled for my annual mammogram. I had recently felt a small lump. It had been coming and going for a few months, but not this month. I never mentioned my suspicions to Tom until after the mammogram. I didn't want to worry him.

The results were quickly in and Tom and I had our worst fear confirmed. Yes, damn! It was BC again. Only it was on the left side this time; so, it wasn't a re-occurrence, but a new case. It turns out that I'd probably been feeling a different lump before. Even so, I still blamed my self.

I met with my surgeon, Dr. Walters, at Allegheny General Hospital on the 27th. I take heart this time, though, as the biopsy showed a type of tubular cancer that stays in situ. There wouldn't be any chemotherapy, just radiation after the standard lumpectomy.

The nurses insist I change and get up on the exam table, but Dr. Walters says that I'm OK where I am sitting in my wheel chair. So he brings my wheelchair over to him, sits opposite me and asked, "How will you get to radiation every weekday, for six weeks?"

My MS had grown worse since I last saw him.

To my great relief, he sensed my distress and suggested a mastectomy rather than a lumpectomy, because then I wouldn't have to submit to radiation. Who'd of thought I'd be so happy.

Tom and I began to feel a little bit optimistic when the wrecking ball swung back again. Dr. Walters begins asking about the fraternal breast cancer that I'd just noted in my medical history update.

I begin telling him about my fraternal aunts, and he gets up and goes to the blackboard, and begins drawing a genealogy chart.

"Yes," I said, in a hyper voice, "two of my dad's sisters, Eloise and Barbara, had BC. Eloise succumbed and died back in the late 60's. My Aunt Barbara has ovarian cancer. And, one of dad's maternal aunts, Winifred Lynch (Figure 6), died from BC."

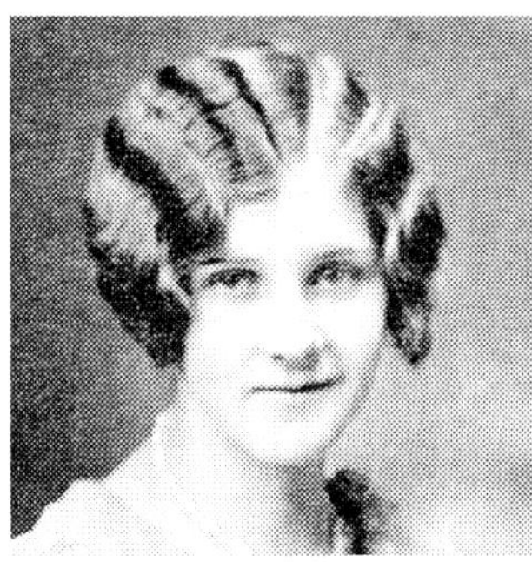

Figure 6 - Winifred Lynch (1911-1976) (Bestowed to Michele Hayes by David Fligger)

Eloise died at age 46 and Winifred was 64 years old when she died. I discovered later that dad's only other sister, Lois, had BC when she was age 50. She has remained cancer free. (See back chart for all.)

Dr. Walters explained that I could be a carrier of the altered and crippled BRCA1, or BRCA2 gene. The BRCA1 gene—it helps control cell division—is a cancer motivator when it doesn't do its job. When the BRCA1 gene is turned "off" it lets the cancer cells run wild. It sounded ominous and ugly, especially, when other genes may be involved that specialists don't know about yet.

It is believed that inherited alterations (called mutations) in the BRCA1 and BRCA2 genes are involved in 30 to 70 percent of all "inherited" cases of breast cancer; the likelihood is highest in families with one or more cases of ovarian cancer.

Note: the percentage risk below is artificially high because studies were done on large families with a mega history of breast cancer. Therefore, the estimates should be considered in a broad range.

BREAST CANCER: 50 to 85 percent (500-850 out of 1000) of women with an altered BRCA1 or BRCA2 gene.

OVARIAN CANCER: 5 to 40 percent (50-400 out of 1000) for women with an altered BRCA1 gene, and 10 to 20 percent (100-200 out of 1000) for women with an altered BRCA2 gene.

If I did the genetic testing and it showed positive for a mutative BRCA1, or BRCA2 gene, should I go one step further and have my ovaries removed like some women have? Would I want to put myself through another operation that could be devastating to my particular form of MS? And, if it ever came to doing the deed, might I propose doing it under twilight, to temper my MS destruction? Well, even though my sense of feeling has diminished, what a wild thought it is.

"In a small but well done study, removal of the ovaries in high–risk women, shows a 70% reduction in breast cancer," said GMA's Dr. Nancy Snyderman, on September 1, 1999.

With MS and BC on dad's side, I appear to be a close genetic link to my fraternal Cousin Lois and her mom, Barbara Nicklow (see back chart). Barbara was diagnosed with BC at the age of 45 and had struggled for ten years with ovarian cancer. In this 1995 interview, for a New Jersey newspaper, she talked about what her artwork represented to her, and how it helped her cope with cancer.

Barbara (Nicklow)...is a remarkable woman and an aspiring artist, who has had ovarian cancer for the last nine years. Barbara has been painting for the last 25 year and expresses her struggle...on canvas. "Art relieves my tension," said Barbara. "My art really helps me express how I feel."

She was once a member of the St. Barnabas Art Group and is presently a member of the Cape May County Art League, Atlantic City Art Center, Society of New Jersey Artists, the National Museum of Women in the Arts in Washington, D.C. and the Ocean City Art Center.

In 1993, Barbara participated in an Ocean City Art Show and it was asked of the artists to paint something personal. "What could be more personal than my cancer?" said Barbara. Barbara created a piece of art that is beautiful in more ways than one. The title of the piece is called, "The Survivor: Before, During and After," in which she faces her past, present and future. The painting displays Barbara sitting at her dressing table brushing her hair and in the mirror she sees herself without hair looking back. On the dressing table is a picture of Barbara, and how she used to be, without the cancer.

After I completed the painting I showed it to my doctor," said Barbara. "After he saw it, he encouraged me to show the painting at the opening of the Joan Karnell Cancer Center in Philadelphia." Barbara took her doctor's advice and displayed her painting at the 1993 opening.

After undergoing four courses of chemotherapy, one course of radiation and five operations, Barbara is overflowing with hope, and plans to never give up her battle with cancer. In her self taught career, Barbara helped design and paint a Victorian Mural in Cape May, served as a judge in several local art shows, and was a board member for the Cape May County Art League for four years. She also assisted artist Cheryl Crews with the Art Career Program at Wildwood Catholic in 1991 and assisted with Teen Art in 1993. She taught drawing class at Cold Spring Village in the summer of 1993 and painted backdrops for several plays. Barbara's paintings are in many private collections in Pennsylvania, New York, New Jersey and Maryland.

Sadly, Barbara passed away on December 26, 1997. She left behind a beautiful legacy.

Having breast cancer twice, and with my interest in genealogy, I now tried harder to dig into the history of my fraternal great grandfather, George Lynch (Figure 7), and his wife, Sarah Catherine Fligger.

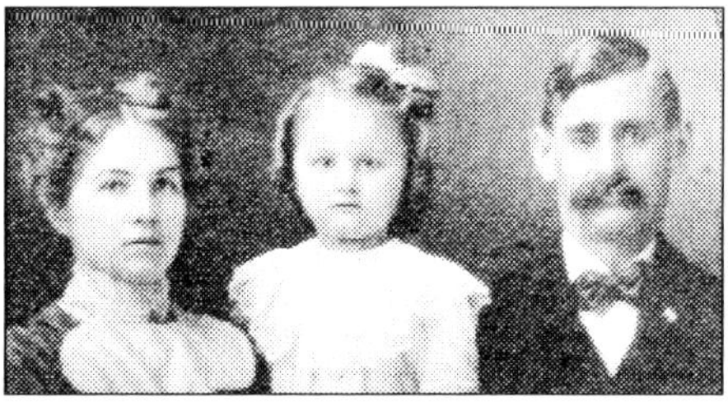

Figure 7 - L to R: Sarah Fligger, Hazel Lynch & George Lynch (Bestowed to Michele Hayes by David Fligger)

My Aunt Lois Nicklow recalls that Sarah's stomach began to swell when she took seriously ill. Did she have cancer—ovarian cancer? I have no information on George and little on Sarah. (See Lynch chart)

Is the Patrick Lynch mentioned in the historical records of Franklin Twp., Fayette County, Pennsylvania (will dated July 25, 1813) related to me?

The family lines of McGuinnis and Shawley a.k.a. Shallus married into the Fligger line. I'm calling all descendants of these specific families. I'm also looking for BC survivors in my Nicklow (Nicola) line.

Genetics is genealogy to the extreme.

Or, perhaps, it was the bad luck of my dad's family that our genes, just suddenly, decided to mutate. Still, it doesn't stop me from screaming, "WHICH ONE OF YOU ANCIENT, DECREPIT, DECEASED CULPRITS GAVE ME THESE ROTTEN GENES?!"

What is there, some genetic time clock, with memory? Has Congress passed a new law? It is hereby understood and agreed that, at the age of forty, "your body shall cruelly and barbarously, strike divers, terrible grievous and dangerous blows to your breast, head and body."

The day came for my surgery on Tuesday, March 17th.

While I was being admitted into Allegheny General, there she was, out of my past, the admitting "Apartment Edie" nurse. I remembered her walk, so I readily recognized her from the back. Anyway, I wish her well now.

Out of surgery, I awoke with absolutely no pain—I took one pain pill just, in case, with a can of pop the nurses gave me. The lack of pain was probably do to nerve damage. Even without the pain or discomfort, they would keep me in for five days due to my dangerous medical history. I was under the care of very attentive and sharp nurses.

To make myself feel better, I decided to wash my hair at the lavatory sink, while one of the nurses changed my bed.

Are you all right?" she asked, rushing over, when I began gasping for breath.

I think the nurses were amazed at me.

The numbness grew worse. I felt its tingly, irritation on the tail end of my spine.

18

A surprise awaited me while I slumbered in my room. Tom was there when my surgeon came in with the news that Friday evening, around 7 o'clock. We had been anxiously waiting for him to show up, since the operation on Tuesday, and couldn't understand why he hadn't stopped in. I guess he didn't have the final biopsy results yet.

He was detached, distantly telling us that the final biopsy, done during the operation, showed positive for the same estrogen-receptor infiltrating ductal carcinoma (IDC) I had had previously. Only this time, it was in least one lymph node.

Dr. Waters said I could do one of three things: I could do nothing, resort to chemo, or.... I was too shocked, at the time, to recall the other, now.

The filthy wrecking ball hammered away again. Oh, what a crushing blow it was. Now, for sure, I had to go through the "purification ritual" of contaminating chemo. Tom phoned his mother right away.

A little while later, after Tom left, Janet called to comfort me and give me support. I babbled on safely keeping an emotional distance.

When I was released from Allegheny General, Tom's mom was nervously waiting for us back at our place with some home made soup for our dinner. Abbey was very excited to see me when we got home.

Two arrangements had been set in place for me through Tom's medical coverage. One was the arrival of a visiting home therapist, who came with more practical advice than I knew; wheelchair ramp angle advice, new exercises for muscle strengthening—by using a thera-band in all sorts of ways, and practical means of transferring.

The one exercise I saw the most benefit from were semi sit-ups, on my long handicap commode, where I could lean back far enough. A soft bed is the choice place for this exercise, because it not only strengths your thigh muscles, but it teaches you better balance.

The second arrangement was a visiting nurse, who stopped in during my "off" chemo weeks. Her name was Beth and a medical supply dropped off any medical equipment that she needed for drawing my blood. If my white count went too low she gave me injections of Leukine that I got from a pharmacy. Of course, she also checked my blood pressure and pulse.

On April 2nd, I visited my oncologist, Dr. Peter Ellis. Now, we had to really decide—was it the chemotherapy drugs, or the Tamoxifen that had caused my cerebral hemorrhage? Dr. Ellis conferred with my neighbor, Dr. Frank Bontempo. They concluded that it had been the Tamoxifen, and I agreed.

Because Dr. Ellis chose the more powerful chemo drug Adriamycin for me, chemo would be just four months, instead of the old six. Caution must be used, though, for it can damage the heart.

So I had my heart checked, on April 10th, through a test they call a MUGA Scan, which stands for "MultiGated blood-pool imaging."

When I phoned for the results, Dr. Madeline Borhani, my devoted and dedicated primary care physician, was dumbfounded and flabbergasted. The MUGA showed a heart that was pumping at only 33%-40%, not the normal 50%-60%.

Its cause was my defective thyroid. Hyperthyroidism gradually makes the heart inefficient, and when left untreated, it can cause congestive heart failure.

I was readily put on the medicines Prinivil and Lanoxin. It was another stumbling block leading back to CMF and six months of treatment.

I struggled through the chemo, making at least a dozen pee trips a day to the bathroom, with extreme fatigue. One side effect started presenting itself, though: a spiking temperature, often at night. Perhaps I had an infection. Calling Dr. Borhani I gave her my suspicions. Yes, a blood test would show positive. And, what was it?

Chemo knocked on the door and gave me menopause.

"Oh, what a nice gift," I sarcastically said, while having a hot flash.

MS'ers certainly know heat isn't compatible with our corroding disease. Our thermostats are broken. So just what am I supposed to do, have an out of body experience?

Nope, no Hormone Replacement Therapy for me, because of my estrogen-receptor driven cancer. Not estrogen, or even natural estrogen, should I consider taking? Does this include such estrogen enhancing food products like soy? Soy is found in tons of processed foods. Even Vitamin E is now encased in soybean oil.

It's been almost two years and I still get "flash sessions" (Tom has so named my hot flashes). When I go through these moments, and because MS can effect breathing, it feels like I'm suffocating or drowning. There's no resonant lung capacity for any commentary screaming.

At the end of my first chemo treatment I was told that I should have a port implanted. It would certainly be less frustrating for the nurses at the oncology office, Beth, and me.

I went in for its insertion on the morning of May 4th. In twilight, I could hear them talking as the surgeon finished.

Later, in outpatient recovery, it was direly clear. The port was not in place. A chest x-ray showed my right lung had been punctured. Usually the neck is tapped for the hookup. In my case, though, the surgeon ventured down toward my lung (which he didn't want to do), because he couldn't find my upper neck-vein. (It was later explained that I have very narrow veins.) They kept me in observation overnight and x-rayed me in the morning.

There was no change. The surgeon decided to insert a tube in my right lung and attach me to a nebulizer. I breathed its moisture along with oxygen. The lung should right itself in short order.

Short order became a retched week. And, every morning they x-rayed.

Because of low white count, and risk of infection, I was given injections of Leukine. The low count probably contributed to the long healing process of my lung.

Since I didn't have full lung capacity, I was to practice deep breathing. On the phone with Janet, the more I tried to catch my breath, the more pain I was in. In agony, I hung up.

Emotionally, I became unfeeling and indifferent. I'd lay in miserable distress, watching the sun set every night, from my private room. But to me there was no sun. It was a slick, shiny black coal of an opaque world and nothing more.

To ease some of the emotional pain, one nurse kindly gave me an evening backrub. Another nurse thought it would be good therapy for me to write my MS story.

"Another local MS sufferer," she said, "has written one. She was a patient here, too."

"Yeah, I read her book," I said.

I don't think it registered to the nurses, how they jump-started me; and snapped me out of my emotional slump. It had to do with the nebulizer.

They kept asking one another, "Should the nebulizer be bubbling, or not, and blah, blah, blah?"

They kept fiddling with it and checking the oxygen gage. That was it!

After they left, I began throwing things from my bed.

I rang the buzzer; "I want to talk to someone who knows what's going on," I demanded.

A little while later in comes the surgeon pushing the portable x-ray machine. I almost expected to see him riding it into the room. Guess I should have screamed sooner.

To make matters worse, I had to retry the port scene. I was released from the hospital on May 11. The procedure had been rescheduled for the 18th. This time the surgeon used a camera to guide him. Chemotherapy resumed the next day. To get through it all I put my mind in isolation.

While I was in the hospital the surgeon asked me why wasn't I furious about it all. Truly, by this time, I was very weary, defeated and tired from "marching with MS, my heart, chemo and cancer—with a hog on my back." Worse than carrying "60 rounds of cartridge in the box gun & knapsacks" was the damn load.

I'm not an angry person in general, and getting upset would just aggravate and stress my MS. I try to conserve energy for any big battle ahead. Burt Lancaster—to maintain stamina in his later years of acting—would sit dormant, until he was called upon to perform.

If there was any benefit to the chemotherapy, I was on for six months, it was the Cytoxan—once used to treat MS symptoms. It seemed to help my inflammation, although it was hard to tell most times. After chemo was over the Cytoxan wonderfully stuck around to enhance my wellbeing, even after a year of being off it. I was able to complete all chemo treatment by October.

Dr. Ellis pronounced me cured. Hurrah!

"My Husband's Brother"

19

On a warm, gorgeous Sunday morning, on October 25, 1998, I telephoned Tom's family, and ask them to join Tom and me in an "end of chemo" celebratory dinner at a local restaurant out in their neighborhood.

I was the only one who hadn't seen Jay (my brother-in-law) since Easter. Everyone close to him had been telling me about his losing weight, and that he looked emaciated and haggard. It was still a shock when I saw him. Due to his diabetes, he'd already had a kidney transplant in November of 1985 and a quintuple heart bypass in 1994.

With a weaker heart by the summer of 1998, (he should have been on a heart transplant list by this time) physicians and specialists weren't optimistic about his future.

After the meal, we all trooped over to his new venture, Cones & Scones, for dessert and ice cream. That was the last time I would to speak to him.

That Monday he slipped into a coma. He laid in the Cannonsburg Hospital for three weeks, trapped between two worlds, before he passed away on November 14th.

Tom spent many evenings at the hospital while I sat at home, alone with my thoughts. I phoned. I wrote. I frantically played computer solitaire, and did my sit-ups with frenzy. The whole time he lay there suffering, I slept with a clenched jaw every night.

I will always remember Jay for his guts and determination.

"A Man of Intestinal Fortitude"

20

Is it possible that some imprinted behavior or genetic character trait can trickle down, from one of our gutsy and determined ancestors, to us? What percentage of our adult buried psyche is rooted in our early childhood experience and upbringing, and how much, if any, is genetic?

"'Behavioral genetics' is a radical revision of contemporary theories of child development, and is fraught with considerable controversy among psychologists."

These researchers have concluded that genetics might have a greater influence on the behavior of children—than was originally thought—and parenting less. They don't claim that heredity is destiny but that "heredity reveals itself through complex interactions with the environment."

Can some unknown spirit lay in wait, inside you, until it deems itself necessary to form a command center? I can be easygoing, or relentless, depending on the need.

Jane Hanna's (Figure 3) brother, Major Alexander Hanna (Figure 5) literally had a wallop of a command center. Here I have used neat details of his life for writing fodder.

Born in 1802, Alexander grew to impressive physical strength, standing six feet and weighing 240 lbs. by age 18. Over his lifetime, it is said he preformed many legendary feats, wrestling men from Harrisburg to Pittsburgh. He once lifted an iron casting weighing 1400 lbs. Another time...

He rode his horse to the Fairall Tavern on the Pennsylvania National Pike (America's first toll road & Route 40 today). A good many loungers were there and to show off his strength, he got under the horse, threw it over a fence and let it lie there until he had attended to his wants in the barroom. In a somewhat similar account Alec picked up a half-grown steer which violently resisted. Effortlessly he slung it about his shoulders and walked away with the animal putting up a fearful howl.

Alexander had a farm located along Hogback Ridge in the Turkeyfoot region of Somerset County. I'm certain he would have been able to carry a "hog on his back" with little effort. And, if he can do it, so can I.

I first heard of Alexander's beating and stabbing from my maternal grandfather, John Beal, and his ma, Annie Harned (Figure 1). Alex had a longstanding feud with the big McClintock family. In May of 1830, five of the McClintock attacked him at a crowded military mustering in Somerset County, Pennsylvania. Upon Alexander's stabbing:

The early reports of this episode describe Dr. Muckenhaupt's surgery as being a half-century in advance of his age. One report, in describing the doctor's skill said, "Muckenhaupt was on hand, sober enough to exercise his keen judgment and wonderful skill." The intestines had collapsed and withered. They were covered with clotted blood and dirt.

The doctor called for a pail of warm water. In this he placed the intestines and gently manipulated them until their circulation and luster were restored. With clean linen cloths he cleaned them. One of the intestines had been entirely severed. He took an ordinary tallow candle, scraped it down to a circumference that accurately fit the caliber of the intestine, slipped both ends of the intestine over the candle so that they met. Then with an ordinary needle and silk thread he united the intestine and sewed up the large wound.

Alexander recovered from his wounds and went on to become a Justice of the Peace in Lower Turkeyfoot Township during the years 1850, 1865, 1872 and 1877. He held a bible in one hand, and with his other hand, he kept a fist.

Everyone is sewn differently and I gather I am too. It's certainly telling, from the very beginning, from the very first paragraph of my story that I wasn't having any newborn fun in the small frame hospital where I was born. There I was a newborn preemie, left in an incubator, without the careful care I needed.

When Mom brought me home she opened tiny unwashed hands. Common sense tells me there had been no close human bonding; and, how could there be with a hospital staff that was probably afraid to handle me.

It wasn't until my mother passed away that my Aunt Patti told me of the hand pinning. I'm sure Mother went on our family doctor's advice concerning my care, and I don't condemn her in any way. I don't want to infer that Mom was a harsh person, because she most assuredly wasn't. She had a soft heart and was tolerant of others, and I loved her very much.

Perhaps because I was singular and isolated at birth, plus the use of hand restraint—these events contributed to my inner strength. This leads me to give some focusing methods that help me keep a positive outlook despite all my troubles. I guess you could call them compartmentalizing, imaging and visualization techniques.

I just don't visualize a crippled nervous system—I think it's a short-circuited electrical system being repaired. I take it further by seeing myself enjoying exciting travel, archaeology, or meeting interesting people. I accomplish this with the help of uplifting "pure moods" music, or sometimes I use pictures.

I've been doing this so-called meditation fantasy for years. It started during my isolated and lonely teen years. No wonder I can be easily hypnotized.

When your mind is uncluttered, open and confident, and you listen to the signals your "spirit" is sending you, warnings of immediate danger may enter your consciousness. Newspaper headlines for my uncanny insight, in the three following stories, might read: "Mysterious Perceptiveness." (Let's not mention Apt. Edie.)

I've labeled these incidents: "ultra" common sense. I believe this gift of intuition had something to do with Mom's common sense habits that she passed on to me. I had forgotten, until now, asking her, "How do you know this or that is right?

"Common sense tells me..." her reply would start.

The following event happened after Tom and I had been married for a few years.

During my usual downtown Pittsburgh lunch hour, I stood waiting to hop a bus out to one of Oakland's medical centers, for a routine allergy injection. The designated bus pulled up, and the back doors sprung open, revealing a lone, black curly haired man, standing with his back to me.

When I started to get on I hesitated, because there was something about him that I questioned. So I went for the front door instead, and all the standing occupants reshuffled with the new passengers. He and I bypassed each other when I moved to the back of the bus.

Then I noticed him out of the corner of my eye, moving back to the rear of the bus again. When he swept by me he whispered something obscene in my ear. I couldn't believe it.

On the return trip to town, he wasn't at my bus stop and I breathed a sigh of relief. Then, like some black comedy, we picked him up at the next stop.

When I got into town, I sneaked out the rear of the bus and went around the back, taking an alternative route to my office building, to make sure that I'd lost him.

A few years ago, another eerie incident occurred when I happened to catch a television show one evening. It showed a husband and wife being interviewed outdoors. They were warmly talking about how much they missed their African home when they were away and how joyful it was to return.

The outdoor television scene showed the husband standing, and speaking wistfully to the camera crew. The sun was shinning through the trees behind him, which gave the scene a sense of longing.

I had an instantaneous thought that he was part of the past. The program host went on to say that lions had mauled him and his wife while they were out walking their grounds.

This other spooky incident occurred during my first year at Penn State. I idolized my Humanities (I) professor, so I signed up for his Humanities (II) class, which met on Tuesdays and Thursdays. A little guy, who was spontaneously and passionately expressive, he hadn't seemed himself lately. I just sat and listened in class, but every once in a while I'd jot down a free-thinking chain of thoughts, in a meager little notebook.

Doing my usual note taking one Thursday, I casually wrote the words "remember this day." It was an odd thing to write and made absolutely no sense when I read it.

Friday night, while I stood in the hall waiting for my ride home, I saw the instructor's wife and dog come in to greet him at the other end of the hall. They had arrived to pick him up. I said "good by" and watched them go out the door.

That was the last time I saw him. I was probably the last student to see him alive. Sadly, that weekend he shot himself.

I hadn't known it at the time, but he had been suffering, and had become despondent, from an inoperable brain tumor. He could no longer get the prescription pain pills he needed, and he couldn't stand the pain any longer.

I kept that "posy" covered meager notepad for years, jotting other notes about life along the way.

I'm not afraid to reveal some of these aspects of myself, nor am I fearful of losing myself. Or, I should say I'm fearless "and" fearful.

For awhile I collected earrings, worried and afraid of losing hand strength and dexterity.

My illness is not who I am. The circumstances of my life are extraneous to who I am. I can dictate and not be a victim if I make a hard enough effort. Paralyzing fear can stop me from moving on towards serenity in life.

When a kid, I awoke to mournful sounds under my bedroom window, late one summer night. I got up the courage and went into my parent's bedroom.

In a voice, quaking with fear, I said to Mom, "There are witches outside my window."

"Go back to bed," she said, "it's just a cat fight."

So I went back to bed.

21

Ever since my second bout with BC, Tom has been saying that I'm due for some good luck and says my upbeat attitude is what keeps him going. But if I give up, so will he. And, without him by my side, I'd probably hang it all up, too.

By turns, I get sad, irritable and moody and Tom gets depressed, too. Frustrated, he wants to corral my troubles. I don't worry for myself, but I worry about the stress on him. I would like to do more of everything for him.

I don't know how Tom puts up with my sudden outbursts, crashing over life's little problems. Sometimes, my anger is not justified and can be hurtful. It's up to me, and it's my choice, whether or not to let some silly, incidental thing, effectively ruin my day, or mar our relationship. I try to catch myself, but I'm bound to slip up somewhere along the line.

Some days I'm frankly cranky and frustrated. Other days I feel blissful.

Tom is an extraordinary guy and a saint. He once went out searching for a fly-by-night barbecue rib place just so I could have a special treat. He always goes out of his way to help anyone who needs it. A lot of men can be insensitive to an ailing spouse, but he makes sure I'm comfortable. He gives such thoughtful love and care, and even though I can be pretty grouchy at times, he has not deserted me.

Tom is always one step ahead of me in the handicap hardware department. One day, he just popped in the house with that wheeled walker. I didn't feel the need for that contraption, but soon enough I was using it. It was the same with the electric wheelchair. I fought him on that one, too. I particularly didn't want a lift on my newer scooter, but eventually found it's great for out-of-reach grocery items at the store.

Depression and sorrow can suddenly come over me like a wave; and, just as suddenly it's gone. Depression is a part of MS. The Nortriptylin I take helps to control my despondency.

The question is are you depressed because you have a chronic illness; or, is it because of demyelination (destruction) in the brain? That's almost impossible to determine; but, in my case—because I seem to have such a good attitude—I'm going to believe it's the latter.

Demyelination in the brain causes dysfunction in memory and cognitive behavior, causing your judgement to be impaired. My day to day memory becomes more of a challenge and I live by routine, calendars and notes on the refrigerator and bathroom mirror. I carry a pen, notepad and caller-ID phone with me in the side pouch of my electric wheelchair at all times. I must be constantly vigilant, which I might add helps keep me mentally alert.

Tom says my personality has changed. The MS, chemo, menopause, the hemorrhage and Grave's disease, have all "monkeyed" with my mind.

MS is beginning to do to my mind what it does to my nervous system. It takes a form of emotional "numbness" and is characterized by my inability to cry, or respond, sometimes. Emotional paralysis is something I've reckoned with lately and at times I feel robbed, empty of myself. I reach out to grasp a fleeting image; what it "feels" like to be my former self, but it always eludes me, like trying to grasp some illusionary apparition.

A very important way I cope with my debilitating disease is humor and I've used it throughout my story. You can especially see this in the following tale.

"Defeated at Gettysburg"

22

Never go anywhere, anytime, on a whim, especially if you have MS. A few summers ago Tom and I drew up a fast plan to visit Gettysburg. We supposed a hotel room would be easily had because we went during the workweek. When we got there, we were so into the lovely day, the historical markers and figuring out the acres of battlefield, that by supper not even a Civil War cot was to be had.

We drove around and around looking for a place. By nightfall—we were heading back towards home by now—we finally found a vacancy. The only glitch was that we'd be bunking with the worst Hells Angels had to offer. Our car lights swept over their lairs, beer and all. When we turned around our car lights also, panned over a car, suspiciously up on blocks. On the way out, paint on a garbage can read "drugs." The "NO" had been obliterated.

Further down the road I saw another place, all lit up.

"Quick, pull over!" I shouted to Tom.

It took us only a minute to realize it was a nursing home.

And a trip up that ugly monstrosity of a lookout tower, the one slated to be demolished on July 3rd, 2000, is more forbidding to the handicapped than Sorbie Tower (ancient, forbidding Hanna stronghold). It was Tom's idea that we stop there first. I could see, staring up at its uninviting presence, that I wasn't in any hurry to go up it.

Like a parody of those two wacky airplane pilots in the comedy *The In–Laws*, the gift shop lady kept going on and on about some instructions, which she then handed to us on a sheet of paper. Leaning over the counter she looked at my scooter.

"Oh, no, that vehicle is much to heavy for the elevator," she absolutely said. “It has to stay below.”

Tom and I were the only two on the elevator, and as it went up we read the bold words: Maximum Weight- 3,000 lbs.

No sooner up, I wailed, "Get me out of here!"

Handicap persons can’t use the usual down elevator, because stairs on the other side access it. Tom ventured down and brought up my scooter, with the key for the same elevator we came up in.

So much for travel light, quick trips. Next time, I’ll have a battle plan.

That’s the thing with a vacation. Should I risk the stress only to end up with a permanent setback? It’s a tradeoff and I no longer seem to recoup what I loose.

A happy homebody, I’ve always been, with a good book, and a cup of tea. Never much of a journeywoman, I’ve always been content to just sit on my perch and gaze out at the pleasant scenery. A vagabond traveler with the world-wondering lust of an Ann Rice vampire—I am not.

"Practical Matters"

23

In my MS case, what worked before now needs practical problem solving, adjusting and reinventing. Tom had to rearrange our master bedroom, because I could no longer use the wall to steady myself. Nor could I reach the closet, or the window blind, without fear of falling. Besides, the chest-of-drawers was in the way.

Tom removed the mirror off our long dresser and moved the dresser in front of our smaller bedroom window, on my side of the bed. He then moved the chest-of-drawers where the dresser had been, now clearing a path for my wheelchair. Finally, he attached a vertical handrail on the side of the heavy dresser, next to me.

For my health, along with daily medicines, I take a multi-vitamin/mineral, 1,000 mg. of Vitamin C, 400 units of Vitamin E and calcium with Vitamin D. A high protein and fiber diet completes the picture. For a little while, I took Evening Primrose oil, which is touted, for the nervous system.

Considering a breast cancer diet, the National Cancer Institute website lists immune enhancing food substances under "Chemoprevention." "This approach involves the use of medication, such as Tamoxifen (except for Michele Hayes) and micronutrients like dietary retinoids and selenium (except for Michele Hayes)."

Selenium, found in whole grains, can trigger allergies in some people, especially in the regions of the United States where selenium is deficient in the soil. The highest food concentrations of this substance—which can be toxic in high doses—are found in Brazil nuts. The very nuts that caused my childhood anaphylaxis. My allergy to nuts I inherited from Mom's side of the family.

There are other MS'ers out there with thyroid problems. I've heard of them. My dad—who may have had Grave's disease—had his thyroid removed when I was two. Could my restless, crazed, childhood activity been attributed to an over-active thyroid? Was I always borderline hyperthyroid?

Do other immune diseases of similar nature link me with anyone in my small, former hometown of Scottdale? A couple of residents in my former neighborhood now have immune conditions, one with lupus and the other with MS.

The girl with lupus grew up next door to me. Could the measles that we shared have been a catalyst—which some experts have said—to our later immune diseases?

Another neighbor across the street eventually died of leukemia. Would investigation show a clustering of immune dysfunction in the neighborhood? I'm sure I'd have heard about it, if it were so.

Enter Montel Williams, on Larry King Live, on August 24, 1999. It was he who proclaimed and exposed, at least for me, the tie between MS and organ deterioration. This is a "call to arms" Montel.

It's a conspiracy! The June 2000 Redbook talks about the new cancer alert for women through released study results. It is an insidious precursor of cancer: breast, ovarian, non-Hodgkin's lymphoma and melanoma.

Yes, it is endometriosis, the autoimmune disease with ravaging cell growth. It doesn't cause cancer but perhaps leads the way. Swedish studies show that women who have it are 30%

more likely to get BC and twice as likely to get OC.

My well–mannered former neurologist, Dr. Benjamin Eidelman, tried to diagnose me with Primary Progressive MS, or Secondary Progressive MS—he wasn't sure which. I didn't neatly fit into a specific category.

He was sharp and attentive, honing right in with keen observation. He gave me answers for a complicated case and identified possible syndromes that I might be enveloped in. Have any other MS'ers been labeled with one or the other of these blood or immune disorders?

The first is Antiphospholipid Antibody Syndrome, a lupus-like syndrome. Thankfully, this was ruled out for me after Dr. Frank Bontempo conducted a study on my blood.

Two more were:

Anticardiolipin Syndrome, is an antibody that is directed against phospholipids, especially the phospholipid cardiolipin and is associated with increased risk for recurring arterial and venous thromboses – also called anticardiolipin in Merriam-Webster's Medical Dictionary, 1995 Edition.

Raynaud's Phenomenon, is a spasm of the superficial blood vessels, especially those of the digits, the fingers and toes. The digits first become cold and pale. Often, the cause...is unknown. It can be brought on by stress. Sometimes, it is a complication of such other conditions as vascular disease, trauma, or disease of the endocrine glands or central nervous system.

Dr. Eidelman, who has since removed to the Florida Mayo Clinic, mentioned the above phenomenon after looking at my badly discolored hands and feet. Because of the Raynaud's, my cold hands may vary from pale translucent to purple, or when hot, to beet red. Raynaud's is secondary to other immune conditions like lupus and rheumatoid arthritis.

At the time I was seeing Dr. Eidelman, I was leery, and so was he, of experimenting with even one of the three ABC drugs: Avonex, Betaseron, and Copaxone, that are currently on the market for MS. The chancy side effects and allergic threats would override any benefit I might glean. I didn't qualify for the latest study here in Pittsburgh. I'm not a candidate for much.

In February 2001, I met with Dr. Galen Mitchell. He's deep into the mystery of MS. Dr. Eidelman, his friend and mentor, drew him to Pittsburgh. I'm in a definite secondary-progressive category, having moved from relapse-remitting. Dr. Mitchell confirmed it after hearing my chronological MS history that I was so aptly to recall and write down. He says that my BC prevents me from taking any of the ABC drugs. He spoke about the new drug Novantrone. It was FDA approved in October 2000, but only for people with normal heart function.

At best, I can barely stand to do my "activities of daily living." Meanwhile, my cold, sometimes inflamed, hands and fingers slowly grow weaker. I plunge them into ice water when they are inflamed. Because of the stroke, my left side is weaker.

I'm becoming hard of hearing; my senses of taste, smell and sight, all have been trampled upon. I have had nystagmus or involuntary eye movement at night. I see a vision pattern forming; spots in front of my eyes, and then the blurring begins. Through my eyes, the colors of life's landscape appear dull and empty.

Am I heading towards dementia? How much is due to the aftereffects of chemo, or menopause, and MS? At times, I feel I'm drifting away, with scattered, fragmented thoughts. I start off listening to conversation and then drift off—somewhere else. Utter drowsiness can garble my words during my attempt at conversation. Going shopping I shake and fumble with mental confusion and indecisiveness.

For the most part, can't remember anything I just read—only how it makes me feel. I haven't gone too far south yet, though, because I've written this (it took me three constant years). I began the manuscript right after my first chemo treatment for my second BC. You can edit writing, but you can't edit "live" talk.

I refuse to have any more mammograms. In the spring of 1999, 2000 and 2001 I had ultra sounds instead. Neither of my breast cancers were spotted through mammograms, even after retake and retake. I found them. Now paranoid, I weekly check for BC.

And, how in the hell are you supposed to sit in a wheelchair with the side of your face plastered against the x-ray machine at a 90° angle? I hear they're trying to come up with a more comfortable test, but still effective.

Another reason I protest is for the sake of the handicap. I'm lucky I have Tom to help me up on the exam table at my tricky OBGYN visits. What about bedridden women with MS who are homebound —what do they do? The Allegheny District Chapter of the NMSS or National Multiple Sclerosis Society is currently addressing these women's health care issues. Magee Women's Hospital is a participant in the in-home clinical exams. (See MS Connection, fall/winter 2000)

My Enterprising Email friend, Mary Palmer, recently sent me a pewter "comfort heart" or "worry heart" from the Breast Cancer Coalition of Rochester, New York. These worry hearts come from Nova Scotia and are created by Oceanart Pewter in Prospect Bay.

A New York woman discovered them, in Oceanart, on her visit back home to Nova Scotia. She and her mother both had breast cancer at the same time, but her mom passed away only after eleven months. The Comfort Heart Initiative, which she set-up, is dedicated in memory of her mother. It is a joint effort between the Canadian Cancer Society and the BCCR to raise funds for research.

I feel genetics will stunningly reveal our past connections with the common ancestors that we all share—with distant peoples and cultures of the world—leading us, perhaps, on a remarkable journey with far reaching implications. Will we be able to trace the birth of breast cancer, multiple sclerosis or other such diseases?

It used to irritate Mom.

I'd excitedly ask her, "You know what?"

"What?" she'd curiously say.

"I don't know," I'd off handily reply.

Today, I'd probably say something like; "It's the spring of 2001. I'm here and I'm cancer free. What a way to welcome in the new millennium. I thank God.

(Aftermath)

On September 19, 1999, the Meadowcroft Rockshelter was dedicated as a historical landmark. Granted by the Pennsylvania Historical and Museum Commission, it was recognized with a "super– sized" blue and yellow plaque.

Presented by Dr. James Adovasio, it represents mankind's pilgrimage in life. It just exemplifies the connection—at least form me—between the cross and all of mankind. Jesus gives "shelter" to all those who seek Him. What a revelation.

Here is part of a splendidly written article, from a local newspaper in southwestern Pennsylvania.

"Celebrating Visitors of the Past:
Meadowcroft Marker Dedicated"

Dr. James Adovasio talks about the Meadowcroft Museum of Rural Life and the prehistoric artifacts discovered below a rockshelter there, like a religious man eager to share his faith.

However, his audience outside the small village's visitors' center Sunday had already been converted. Most of the 35 people who sat on folding chairs or stood in the hot afternoon sunshine already knew the rockshelter represents the oldest dated and longest continually used human site in North America. They have closely followed the work of Adovasio and his teams of archaeologists over the past 26 years and understand the ramifications of all that they have unearthed.

"What we celebrate today is all those who passed this way and left their traces on the path," said Adovasio, principal investigator of the rockshelter....

Descendants of George Lynch

1 **George Lynch** b: abt. 1880 in PA?
+**Sarah "Sadie" Catherine Fligger** b: 9-15-1882 at Westmoreland Co., PA **(DIED CANCER ?)**
2 **Hazel Mary Lynch** b: 12-6-1902 at Hunker, E. Huntingdon Twp., West. Co., PA
+**Quincy Hixon Nicklow** b: 1-18-1897 at Ruffsdale, E. Huntingdon Twp., West. Co., PA
3 **George D. Nicklow** d: infancy?
3 **Pearl Eloise Nicklow** b: 4-1-1923 at Ruffsdale, E. Huntingdon Twp., West. Co., PA **(DIED OF BC, AGE 45)**
3 **Quincy Quay "Nick" Nicklow** b: 2-17-1926 at Ruffsdale, E. Huntingdon Twp., West. Co., PA **(CEREBRAL HEMORAGE, DIED AGE 40)**
+Jeanne Audrey Beal
4 **Michele Quay "Shelley"** **(MS,BC,CEREBRAL HEMORAGE)**
+Thomas Plynn Hayes, Jr.
3 **Lois Jean Nicklow** b: 3-11-1929 at Ruffsdale, E. Huntingdon Twp., West. Co., PA **(BC AGE 50)**
3 **James Donald Nicklow** b: 12-7-1930 at Ruffsdale, E. Huntingdon Twp., West. Co., PA
3 **Barbara Nicklow** b: 1-29-1935 at Ruffsdale, E. Huntingdon Twp., West. Co., PA **(BC, AGE 45 — DIED OF OC, AGE 60)**
+William Knipple
4 **Patricia Knipple**
+Unknown
5 **Daughter (GRAVE'S DISEASE)**
4 **Lois Knipple (MS; TYPE 2 DIABETES)**
3 **Lawrence Richard Nicklow** b: 7-13-1939 at Ruffsdale, E. Huntingdon Twp., West. Co., PA **(DIED LUNG CANCER)**
2 **Fred Lynch** b: Aft. 12-6-1902
2 **Harry Lynch** b: Aft. 12-6-1902
2 **Irene Lynch** b: Aft. 12-6-1902
2 **Janet Lynch** b: Aft. 12-6-1902
2 **Winifred Lynch** b: 11-6-1911 at Hunker, E. Huntingdon Twp., West. Co., PA **(DIED BC, AGE 64)**
2 **Frank Lynch** b: 7-16-1913 at Hunker, E. Huntingdon Twp. , West. Co., PA. **(DIED ALZHEIMER'S DISEASE)**

Descendants of Mary McGinnis

1 **Mary McGinnis** b: 11-20-1807 at Mt. Pleasant Twp., West. Co., PA d: 7-7-1870 Donegal, Donegal Twp., West. Co., PA

+Samuel Fligger b: 2-4-1807 d: 2-15-1888 at Donegal, Donegal Twp., West. Co., PA

2 **David M. Fligger** b: 6-26-1836 at Donegal Twp., Westmoreland Co., PA d: 1910, Donegal Twp., West Co., PA

+Margaret L. Shawley (SHALLUS) b: ABT 1853 at Jones Mills, West. Co., PA d: 1913

3 **Sarah "Sadie" Catherine Fligger** b: 9-15-1882 at Westmoreland Co., PA **(DIED CANCER?)**

+George Lynch b: abt. 1880 in PA?

Family of J. B. Hanna, Sr., Honorable

1 **James B. Hanna, Sr., Honorable (5th GGrandfather)**
+Ann Leech
2 John "Judge" Hanna, Honorable
2 Mary Hanna
2 Thomas Hanna
2 James B. Hanna, Jr.
2 **Alexander Hanna, Major**
2 William "Uncle Billy" Hanna
2 Phoebe Hanna
2 **Jane Hanna (4th GGrandmother)**
2 Martha Hanna
2 Anne Hanna

Footnotes and References

Emmylou Harris, *Wrecking Ball*, New York: Electra Entertainment Group, a Division of Time Warner, Inc., 1995.

J. M. Adovasio, J.D. Gunn, J. Donahue, and R. Stuckerrath, "Excavation at Meadowcroft Rockshelter, 1973-1974: A Progress Report," *Pennsylvania Archaeologist*, Vol. 44, No. 3, September 1975, page 1.

Ibid.,page, 15.

Thomas Y. Canby, " Search for the First Americans," *National Geographic*, September 1979, pages 354-355.

Ibid.

Michael Parfitt, "Hunt for the First Americans," *National Geographic*, December 2000, pages 41-67.

Ibid.

L R Beatty, (Adapted from a story by Gilbert Love), "Story of the Great Cross," *Jumonville...A Premier Camp, Conference, and Retreat Center*, http://www.gospelcom.net/cci/jumonville/textonly/general/jcross.html

Thomas R. Hester, Editor, "Introduction," *An Archaeological Survey of the Radium Springs Area, Southern New Mexico*, Center for Archaeological Research The University of Texas at San Antonio, 1977.

Stephen L. Black, (Thomas R. Hester-Editor) "Archaeological Background," *An Archaeological Survey of the Radium Springs Area, Southern New Mexico*, Center for Archaeological Research The University of Texas at San Antonio, 1977, page 26.

Susan Ince, "The New Cancer Risk," *Redbook*, June 2000, page 47.

WebMD, http://my.webmd.com/content/dmk/dmk_article_40061

Ibid.

E. Howard Blackburn, History of Bedford and Somerset Counties, Vol. 1, 1906, NY.

Emmylou Harris, *Wrecking Ball*, New York: Electra Entertainment Group, a Division of Time Warner, Inc., 1995.
http://www.nolvadex.com/facts.asp

"Graves' Disease," *Mayo Clinic Health Education*, http://www.mayohealth.org/mayo/pted/htm/graves.htm

National Cancer Institute,
http://cancernet.nci.nih.gov/clinpdq/risk/Genetic_Testing_for_Breast_Cancer_Risk:__It's_Your_Choice.html

"Erma's Barbara Knipple Battles Cancer With Art," *Lower Township Gazette*, November 24, 1995.

US GenWeb, Fayette County, Pennsylvania , ftp://ftp.rootsweb.com/pub/usgenweb/pa/fayette/history/local/early-sett01.txt

August Sessions, No. 4, Somerset Co. Courthouse, 1830.
http://www.advocatehealth.com/healthinfo/articles/heartcare/noninvase/mugascan.html

Annie Murphy Paul, "Kid Stuff: Do Parents Really Matter?" *Psychology Today*, February 1988, page 46.

Ibid., page 46.

Michael P. Connelly, "Alexander Hanna: Strength of Body and Character," *Laurel Messenger*, May 1996, pages 1-3.

Ibid., page 2.

http://www.friendsofgettysburg.org/

National Cancer Institute,
http://cancernet.nci.nih.gov/clinpdq/risk/Genetic_Testing_for_Breast_Cancer_Risk:__It's_Your_Choice.html

Susan Ince, "The New Cancer Risk," *Redbook*, June 2000, pages 46 & 47.

WebMD, http://my.webmd.com/content/c4_asset/merriam-webster_medical_dictionary_144558

WebMD, http://my.webmd.com/content/dmk/dmk_article_1459185

"Celebrating Visitors of the Past," *The Observer*, September 1999.